The Beginner's
PEGAN
DIET
COOKBOOK

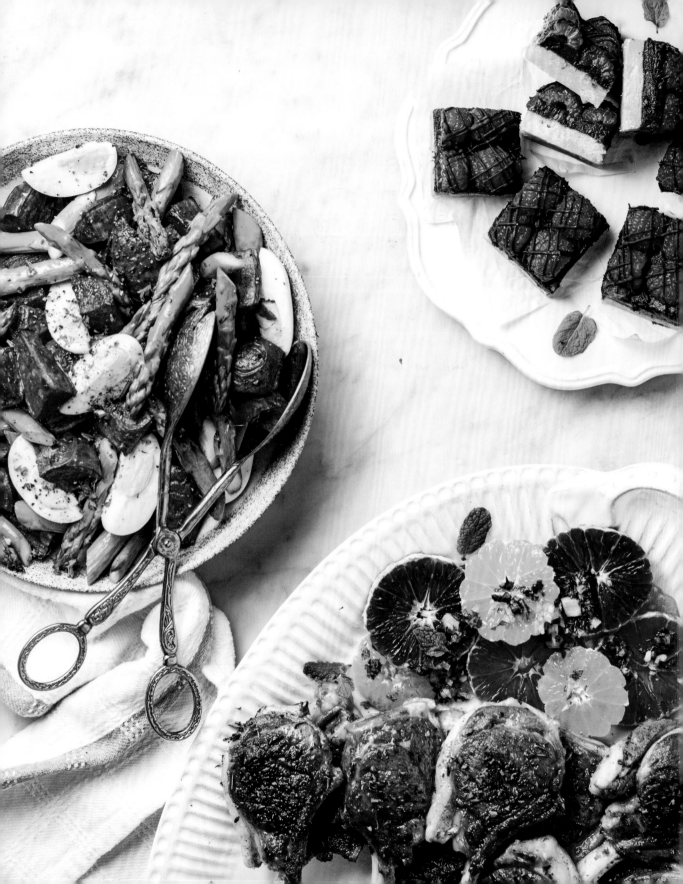

The Beginner's
PEGAN
DIET
COOKBOOK

Plant-Forward Recipes Combining the Best of the **PALEO** and **VEGAN** Diets for Lifelong Health

MICHELLE MILLER

FAIR WINDS

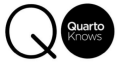

Inspiring | Educating | Creating | Entertaining

Brimming with creative inspiration, how-to projects, and useful information to enrich your everyday life, Quarto Knows is a favorite destination for those pursuing their interests and passions. Visit our site and dig deeper with our books into your area of interest: Quarto Creates, Quarto Cooks, Quarto Homes, Quarto Lives, Quarto Drives, Quarto Explores, Quarto Gifts, or Quarto Kids.

First Published in 2021 by Fair Winds Press, an imprint of The Quarto Group, 100 Cummings Center, Suite 265-D, Beverly, MA 01915, USA.
T (978) 282-9590 F (978) 283-2742 QuartoKnows.com

Fair Winds Press titles are also available at discount for retail, wholesale, promotional, and bulk purchase. For details, contact the Special Sales Manager by email at specialsales@quarto.com or by mail at The Quarto Group, Attn: Special Sales Manager, 100 Cummings Center, Suite 265-D, Beverly, MA 01915, USA.

25 24 23 22 21   1 2 3 4 5

ISBN: 978-1-59233-946-4
Digital edition published in 2021
eISBN: 978-1-63159-875-3

Library of Congress Cataloging-in-Publication Data

Names: Miller, Michelle, author.
Title: The beginner's pegan diet cookbook : plant-forward recipes combining the best of the paleo and vegan diets for lifelong health / Michelle Miller.
Other titles: Pegan diet cookbook
Description: Beverly, MA : Fair Winds Press, 2021. | Includes index. | Summary: "The Beginner's Guide to the Pegan Diet offers guidance and 100+ amazing recipes for this balanced, anti-inflammatory blend of the paleo and vegan diets"-- Provided by publisher.
Identifiers: LCCN 2020039716 (print) | LCCN 2020039717 (ebook) | ISBN 9781592339464 (trade paperback) | ISBN 9781631598753 (ebook)
Subjects: LCSH: High-protein diet--Recipes. | Vegan cooking. | Cooking (Natural foods) | LCGFT: Cookbooks.
Classification: LCC RM237.65 .M54 2021 (print) | LCC RM237.65 (ebook) | DDC 641.5/638--dc23
LC record available at https://lccn.loc.gov/2020039716
LC ebook record available at https://lccn.loc.gov/2020039717

Design: Megan Jones Design
Page Layout: Megan Jones Design
Photography: Michelle Miller

Printed in China

The information in this book is for educational purposes only. It is not intended to replace the advice of a physician or medical practitioner. Please see your health-care provider before beginning any new health program.

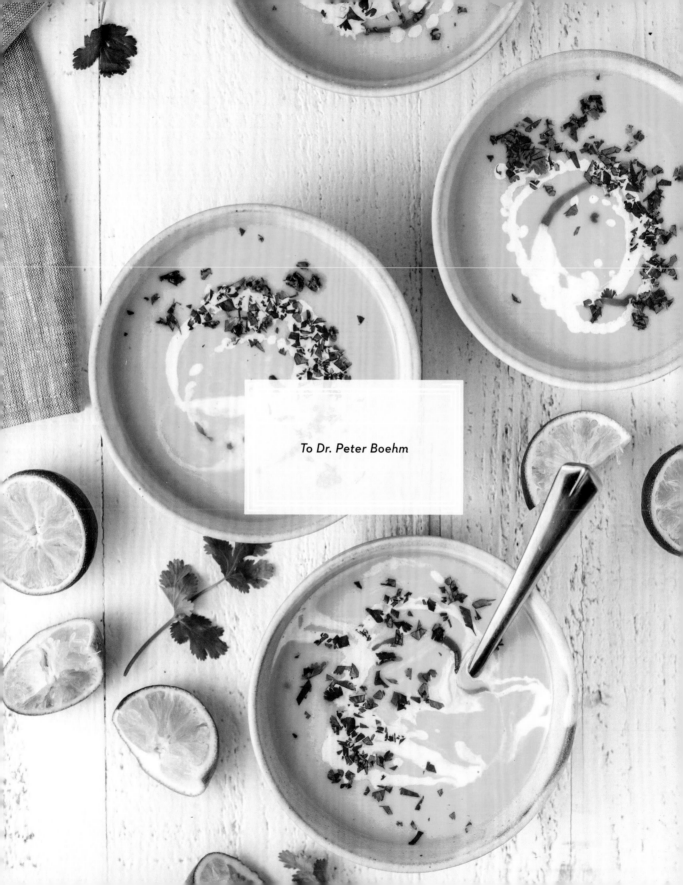

To Dr. Peter Boehm

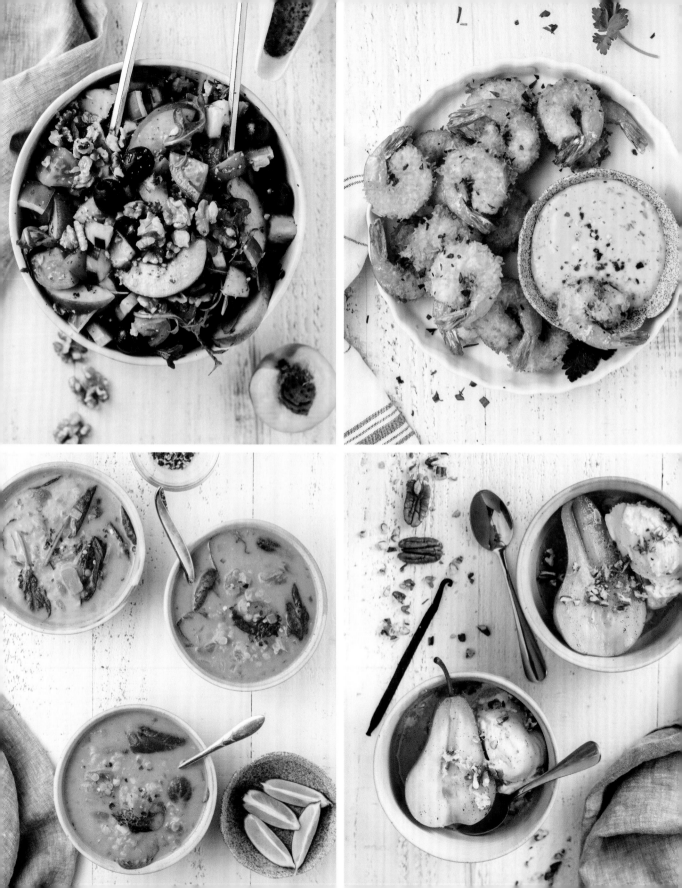

CONTENTS

INTRODUCTION

◇ ◇ ◇

When I was young, I was sick and unhealthy. I was diagnosed with exercise-induced asthma at the age of six and, from that point on, was on steroid inhalers and often prescribed steroids to make it through bouts of bronchitis. At the age of twelve, I was overweight and rarely slept through the night without waking up needing to use my inhaler.

That winter, my regular doctor was away, and I saw Dr. Peter Boehm, a man who had the most profound impact on the rest of my life. He looked at my records and explained that the repeated rounds of steroids were a bandage, but not addressing the root cause of my illness. Instead of looking at the illness I was dealing with, he looked at me as a twelve-year-old, otherwise healthy child, and knew he needed to do a little investigating.

In the course of two days, we found out I had many airborne allergies. He recommended that my mom remove the carpet from my room and bleach my walls to get rid of any mold. That night, for the first night in as long as I could remember, I slept solidly, without needing medication.

Being able to sleep through the night gave me levels of energy I hadn't experienced before. I started running at school with a friend and joined a gym. As the weight started coming off, I became interested in health, fitness, and nutrition and found ways to add more whole foods to my diet.

At that first appointment, Dr. Boehm told me we were going to figure this out and, one day, I would send him a postcard telling him about the marathon I just ran. That encouragement has stuck with me for more than twenty years now. I have run half-marathons and am now training for a full marathon.

The heart of the pegan diet is to understand the whole person and how our choices affect our health in so many ways. I am so grateful to have met Dr. Boehm, who looked at me as a whole person and helped put me on track for a healthy and full adulthood.

"THE HEART OF THE PEGAN DIET IS TO UNDERSTAND THE WHOLE PERSON AND HOW OUR CHOICES AFFECT OUR HEALTH IN SO MANY WAYS."

CHAPTER 1

◆ ◆ ◆

THE BASICS OF THE PEGAN DIET

The science of food and nutrition is ever changing and understanding what we should eat and why is a never-ending quest. Experts have been influenced by food manufacturers turning what should be science-based advice into heavily political topics.

INTRODUCTION

Dietary advice has vastly changed over the past seventy-five years. In the 1950s, we were told that cholesterol was bad for us and to limit fats and animal products. This brought on heavily grain-based diets full of processed foods. Instead of helping, this bolstered the obesity epidemic, skyrocketing cases of diabetes with nearly fifteen times the number of cases in 2017 compared to 1958.

It's time to recognize the flaws in our health care and education systems. We've been given bad advice, but the truth about food is within our grasp.

Food comes from the earth. In its purest state, it is whole and natural. Convenience foods, processed foods, and fast foods have very little place in a healthy, functional diet. Dr. Mark Hyman, functional medicine doctor and creator of the pegan diet, reminds us that if it comes with a label, we probably shouldn't eat it.

Understanding which foods provide our bodies with disease-fighting nutrients, and which foods provide little nutritional value, clarifies what belongs on our plates.

The *pegan* (coined from a combination of the paleo and vegan diets) diet is a blend of the healthiest aspects of paleo and vegan diets without the firm restrictions those diets demand. It goes beyond just the nutrition of food, exploring how choosing organic, sustainable, and ethical meats and produce are better for our planet and our bodies.

AN OVERVIEW OF DR. MARK HYMAN'S PEGAN DIET PRINCIPLES

The pegan diet focuses on real, whole foods, and prioritizes the most nutrient-dense options. It is centered on fueling the body with high-quality foods: meats, low-carbohydrate fruits and vegetables, nuts, and seeds. These foods provide the highest nutrient content with the least impact on blood sugar levels. Although gluten is avoided on this diet, gluten-free grains are allowed in moderation along with legumes, healthy full-fat dairy products, and low glycemic sweeteners.

At the core of this diet is a lifestyle that takes into account optimal health as well as recognizing the need for environmentally sustainable food and animal welfare.

Understanding which foods to avoid is equally important.

AVOID OR LIMIT

- Artificial sweeteners
- Dried fruits, such as figs and raisins, that have a very high glycemic index
- Food additives and preservatives
- Gluten-containing grains
- Oils high in omega-6 fatty acids, such as corn, cottonseed, soybean, and sunflower
- Processed grain foods, such as bread, cereals, and crackers
- Processed sugars
- Trans fats (hydrogenated oils)

UNDERSTANDING THE GLYCEMIC INDEX

Optimal health is at the core of the pegan diet. The medical community's current understanding of how glycemic load affects our health is a driving factor in determining how to fuel our bodies.

Foods with a high glycemic load, such as processed grain foods, potatoes, and sugar, spike blood sugar levels, leading to inflammation. Unstable blood sugar levels cause diabetes and contribute to heart disease and some types of cancer.

The glycemic index of a food is determined by how much that food raises your blood sugar level compared to pure glucose. The glycemic load refers to how much a typical serving of a food raises your blood sugar level. So, although watermelon has a glycemic index of eighty, its glycemic load is only five, making it a good food choice.

Focusing the majority of your diet on low glycemic–load foods helps control blood sugar levels, which makes it easier to maintain or lose weight, wards off health issues, and leads to more stable energy levels.

WHAT SHOULD WE EAT?

Although the pegan diet is described as a combination of vegan and paleo diets, I like to think of it as a plant-forward paleo diet with allowances for healthier nonpaleo foods, such as gluten-free grains, legumes, and fermented dairy products.

Plant foods, such as low glycemic fruits and vegetables, nuts, and seeds, are the most nutrient-dense options, so they should make up most of our plates. Animal proteins provide nutrients of a quality not found in plant foods and are vital to our health.

Fruits and Vegetables

A key consideration when choosing fruits and vegetables is glycemic index. Options that significantly raise blood sugar are detrimental to our health, causing food cravings and inconsistent energy levels throughout the day. This leads to overeating and lowers self-control when it comes to choosing the right foods to fuel our bodies.

LOW GLYCEMIC FRUITS

Fruit should be eaten in moderation based on your health and goals. People who are diabetic, prediabetic, or struggle to maintain a healthy weight should consider avoiding fruit or sticking to low-carbohydrate berries.

A general rule is to include one to three servings of fruit per day.

Fruit makes a great snack. Pair berries with dark chocolate and nuts or a piece of citrus with cut vegetables and dip. Pomegranate, avocado, and stone fruit make excellent additions to salads and even meat dishes at meals. If using fruit in smoothies, be sure to include veggies, whole milk yogurt, and healthy fats to keep the overall sugar content low.

Avoid high glycemic–load fruits such as bananas and dried fruits such as figs, dates, and raisins.

LOW GLYCEMIC FRUITS

- Apple
- Avocado
- Berries, such as blackberries, blueberries, cranberries, elderberries, goji berries, raspberries, and strawberries
- Citrus, such as grapefruit, lemons, limes, mandarins, and oranges
- Grapes
- Guava
- Kiwi
- Mango
- Melon, such as cantaloupe, honeydew, and watermelon
- Pears
- Pineapple
- Pomegranate
- Stone fruit, such as apricots, nectarines, peaches, and plums

LOW GLYCEMIC VEGETABLES

- Artichokes
- Asparagus
- Bell pepper
- Broccoli
- Broccoli rabe
- Brussels sprouts
- Carrot
- Cauliflower
- Cucumber
- Eggplant
- Fennel
- Greens, such as arugula, cabbage, chard, collard greens, dark-colored lettuce, kale, spinach, and watercress
- Herbs, such as basil, chives, cilantro, and parsley
- Mushrooms
- Okra
- Onion
- Parsnip
- Radish
- Sprouts
- Tomato
- Turnip and turnip greens
- Winter squash, such as butternut, delicata, and pumpkin
- Zucchini

LOW GLYCEMIC VEGETABLES

Vegetables will become your best friends on the pegan diet. To beat boredom, experiment with vegetables you haven't tried before like maybe broccoli rabe or fennel. Build salads around a variety of greens, throw a colorful mix onto a sheet pan to roast, and keep veggies for stir-fries stocked at all times. Eating a variety of raw and cooked vegetables and using interesting sauces and dressings will keep things fresh.

Nuts and Seeds

Nuts and seeds are another great source of nutrition, healthy fats, and proteins. Although high in calories, they provide nutrients such as zinc and magnesium, and have anti-inflammatory polyunsaturated fats, monounsaturated fats, and omega-3s. Combined with a high fiber content, they are nutritional powerhouses that aid weight loss, help prevent type 2 diabetes, and lower the risk of heart disease and cancer.

NUTS AND SEEDS TO HAVE ON HAND

- Almonds
- Cashews
- Chia seeds
- Flaxseed
- Hemp seeds
- Macadamia nuts
- Pecans
- Pistachios
- Pumpkin seeds
- Sesame seeds
- Sunflower seeds
- Walnuts

Plus, they are delicious and portable. Nuts are a great snack to take on the go or for powering up for physical activity. I often snack on nuts when I know a meal is an hour or more away.

Instead of croutons on salads or soups, try a sprinkling of nuts or toasted seeds for a burst of nutrition and a little crunch and flavor. Instead of bread crumbs, coat your veggies or meats with ground nuts, like pistachios or almonds, for a flavorful, crunchy texture.

Peanuts are not nuts—they are legumes and are not the healthiest choice.

Legumes

Although legumes do contain higher amounts of protein than other plants, they are still low in protein compared to animal products.

Beans are best enjoyed in moderation. Adding them to salads or soups is a great way to add fiber to your meals. However, a diet heavy in beans can cause digestive issues as well as add unneeded starch.

A good rule is to enjoy ¼ to ½ cup (weight varies) of beans with several meals a week rather than making them a daily staple.

LEGUMES TO ENJOY IN MODERATION

- Black beans
- Chickpeas
- Kidney beans
- Lentils

THE BEST SOURCES OF MEATS, POULTRY, EGGS, SEAFOOD, DAIRY, AND CONDIMENTS

Although protein is found in many plant foods, eggs, meat, poultry, and seafood are the best sources of protein for a healthy, low glycemic diet.

Previous advice to avoid red meat or egg yolks in your diet to lower saturated fat intake has been debunked and, although a solid recommendation for a level of saturated fat to include hasn't been reached, it's now being seen as neutral, rather than positive or detrimental to our health.

Though plant foods contain protein, especially legumes and some whole grains, there aren't many plants that contain all the essential amino acids our bodies need, which means they aren't *complete* proteins. Buckwheat and quinoa contain complete proteins, but you must consume large amounts of beans and grains to equal the protein found in small portions of beef, pork, poultry, or seafood.

In addition, these foods are the only sources of vitamin B_{12} and contain high amounts of certain nutrients, such as B vitamins, iron, and vitamins D and E, and minerals such as magnesium, potassium, selenium, sodium, and zinc. Meat is, essentially, the original superfood.

Unfortunately, modern meat-raising practices have altered the animals' natural diets. We are feeding the animals grains rather than grasses and grubs and have turned to hormone use and antibiotics to increase the animals' weights. As a result, conventionally raised animals are much less nutritious than organic, grass-fed, or pastured animals.

It's important to consider how the animals are fed, whether they are being raised humanely, and the environmental impact of farming practices. Following is an explanation of how to choose the best animal products based on these concerns.

Beef and Lamb

Purchasing and consuming meats raised naturally have a big impact on their nutritional value. Conventionally raised animals are fed grains to fatten them up quickly and cheaply. Unfortunately, they are also given hormones and antibiotics that speed the maturation of the animals. This is done without regard for the nutrition of the animals or how it affects us when we consume them.

One of the most convincing arguments for choosing grass-fed and pastured meats is their increased omega-3 content. Our bodies need a higher ratio of omega-3 to omega-6 fatty acids. The standard American diet (SAD) is heavy on grains and seed oils, which are high in omega-6s. This skewed ratio causes inflammation. Grass-fed and pastured meats have five times the omega-3 content, helping push this ratio in a healthier direction.

The fats in grass-fed meats are also rich in conjugated linoleic acids (CLAs), containing up to 500 percent more CLAs than grain-fed meat and dairy products. These powerful fatty acids are only found in a few foods, and grass-fed butter and meat are the best sources of CLAs.

CLAs have been proven to slow the growth of cancerous tumors as well as reduce the risk of heart disease and diabetes. Diets high in CLAs are also attributed to weight control and higher metabolism.

Besides the overwhelming nutritional superiority, grass-fed animals are more humanely treated, often having outdoor space to roam and forage. Conventionally raised cows are given several months to live outdoors before being forced into feedlots where space is limited. The animals are injected with hormones and antibiotics, making the meat less safe and more susceptible to disease than naturally raised meat.

Poultry and Eggs

Chicken, duck, and turkey eggs are also great sources of protein, but there are many factors to consider when purchasing them.

According to Dr. Hyman, 90 percent of chickens consumed in the United States are raised on concentrated animal feeding operations (CAFOs), where they are continually injected with antibiotics to contain the spread of diseases in these highly crowded spaces.

Conventionally raised birds are sometimes given less than one square foot to live in, meaning they grow faster due to less activity. Living on top of their own waste causes the spread of diseases such as salmonella.

Free-range birds are allowed to spend at least half their lives outside, foraging for grass, which provides them access to a natural diet.

To ensure your poultry and eggs are as healthy as possible, look for pastured eggs and poultry. This means the animals are truly free-range and have access to a natural diet rather than being fed GMO soy- and corn-based foods.

Pastured chickens have higher omega-3s and more antioxidants due to their grass-based diet.

Pastured eggs have twice the amount of omega-3s plus more vitamins D and E, and beta-carotene.

Even pastured chicken has a high omega-6 to omega-3 ratio, so balance your diet with omega-3-rich options, such as grass-fed beef and wild seafood.

Seafood

There are two issues of concern when it comes to incorporating seafood into your diet: mercury content and whether the fish is wild or farm raised.

Pollution in our oceans has led to high amounts of mercury being consumed by marine life. The mercury is concentrated as it passes from one organism to another, meaning animals high on the food chain have higher levels of mercury contamination.

Smaller fish, such as anchovies and sardines, have the lowest levels of mercury. Salmon has a moderate level. Larger fish, such as ahi tuna, shark, and swordfish, have the highest levels of mercury.

Although seafood is still part of a nutritious diet, limiting consumption of larger fish to once a week is good practice.

Regarding the second issue—purchasing wild versus farmed fish—farmed fish are often raised in crowded confines, meaning they are exposed to pollutants and toxic contaminants at a much higher rate than wild seafood.

Wild seafood eat a natural diet whereas farm-raised fish eat a high-fat feed made of corn, grain, and fish meal. This low-cost feed fattens up the fish quickly, but the cost to the consumer is a less nutritious fish.

Reap the benefits seafood does offer by choosing wild-caught seafood and incorporating more small fish into your diet.

Dairy

Dairy products, as a whole, are difficult for most adults to digest. *Healthline* reports that 75 percent of adults are lactose intolerant, which can lead to acne, allergies, asthma, bloating, eczema, gas, and irritable bowel syndrome (IBS).

Some exceptions to this rule exist, such as for fermented dairy products and butter.

DAIRY PRODUCTS TO ENJOY IN MODERATION

- Goat cheese or raw cheese
- Grass-fed butter
- Grass-fed ghee
- Plain kefir
- Plain yogurt

Oils, Vinegars, and Condiments

Oils, vinegars, and condiments are a great way to add flavor and nutrition to the foods we eat. Choosing the best ones often comes down to choosing the simplest options.

OPT FOR UNREFINED OILS HIGH IN MONOUNSATURATED FATS

- Avocado oil
- Coconut oil
- Macadamia nut oil
- Olive oil
- Walnut oil

Vinegars are great for adding a splash of flavor to foods as well as aiding digestion and helping improve nutrient absorption.

MY FAVORITE VINEGARS TO STOCK

- Apple cider vinegar
- Balsamic vinegar
- Red wine vinegar
- Rice wine vinegar
- White wine vinegar

Other condiments are more difficult to navigate. Most mainstream store-bought options have added sugars, chemicals, and preservatives that make them less than ideal choices. When possible, opt for homemade condiments made from simple, clean ingredients.

CONDIMENTS TO AVOID

- Barbecue sauce, which is loaded with sugar
- Ketchup made with high fructose corn syrup
- Mayonnaise made with refined vegetable oils high in omega-6 fatty acids
- Salad dressings with refined oils, sugars, or preservatives
- Soy sauce made with GMO soybeans and wheat

CONDIMENTS TO ENJOY

- Coconut aminos, a natural alternative to soy sauce
- Hot sauces, especially those made without gums or preservatives
- Mayonnaise made with avocado oil
- Mustard, especially types with no added sugars
- Nut butters (Prioritize those made with only nuts and salt; avoid those made with refined oils and sugars.)

The Evolution of Grains and Their Place in Our Diet

The most popular foods in Western diets are also some of the most detrimental to our health. Corn, wheat, and white rice are avoided on the pegan diet, not only because they are less nutritious and have high glycemic loads but also because the agricultural practices used to grow these crops are devastating to our environment. The mass production of these crops consumes a lot of resources, including water, fossil fuels, and fertilizers.

Wheat is particularly concerning because it contains gluten. Although only a small percentage of the population has celiac disease or is allergic to gluten, studies have shown that gluten damages the gut—even in people who show no other signs of intolerance.

Some gluten-free grains are included in the pegan diet. Because all grains raise blood sugar levels, restrict consumption to two or three ½-cup (weight varies) servings per week and avoid them completely if you're diabetic or struggle to lose or maintain weight.

GLUTEN-FREE GRAINS TO INCORPORATE IN YOUR DIET

- Amaranth
- Buckwheat
- Millet
- Quinoa
- Rice: black, brown, red, or wild

Sugars and Sweeteners

Although following the pegan diet, generally, means restricting or avoiding sweeteners, there are allowances for low glycemic sweeteners.

Avoid artificial sweeteners made from chemicals. These sweeteners aren't safe for consumption. They can lead to intestinal distress and have been shown to cause cancer in lab animals. Look for and avoid additives such as acesulfame potassium, aspartame, neotame, saccharin, and sucralose.

HIGH GLYCEMIC SWEETENERS TO AVOID

- Brown sugar
- Granulated table sugar
- Syrups made with refined sugars

NATURAL SWEETENERS WITH LOWER GLYCEMIC LOADS TO ENJOY IN MODERATION

- Coconut sugar
- Date sugar
- Honey
- Maple syrup
- Monk fruit
- Stevia

THE 75 PERCENT/ 25 PERCENT PLATE

For optimal health, the foods on your plate should focus on the most nutrient-rich foods, like low glycemic index vegetables and fruit.

The next thing to add to a healthy plate is a quality source of protein. Vary proteins in meals throughout the week but be sure to add wild, low-mercury seafood and grass-fed beef or lamb. These are the best sources of omega-3s that are needed to keep a healthy omega-6 to omega-3 ratio. Meat contains all essential amino acids in quantities superior to protein-rich plant foods and the proteins are more bioavailable. Most meals need to contain meat, poultry, eggs, or seafood for adequate protein. A healthy portion of meat is 4 to 6 ounces (115 to 170 g) per meal for an adult.

Healthy fats, such as avocado; anti-inflammatory oils, such as avocado, coconut, and olive; and nuts and seeds should be included in small to moderate quantities. Fats are needed to help the body absorb the fat-soluble vitamins—A, D, E, and K—found in plant foods. The body uses fats to help regulate hormones, signal hunger, regulate body temperature, and construct cell membranes.

Use these plates as an example of how to build meals that provide our bodies with energy and all the key nutrients needed to thrive:

PLATE 1

- 2 cups (40 g) arugula
- 2 tablespoons (22 g) pomegranate arils
- 2 tablespoons (14 g) pecans
- 1 tablespoon (15 ml) olive oil–based salad dressing
- 1 cup (124 g) roasted or steamed cauliflower
- One 4-ounce (115 g) roasted salmon fillet

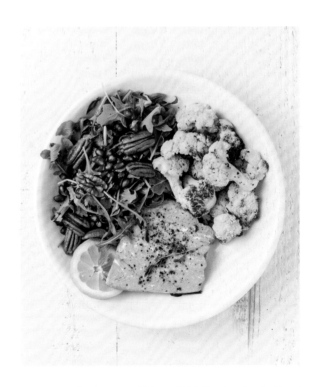

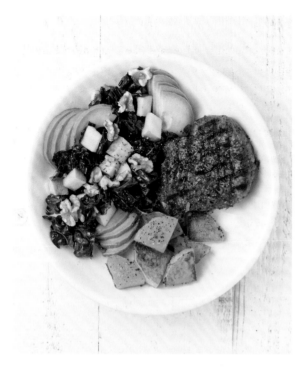

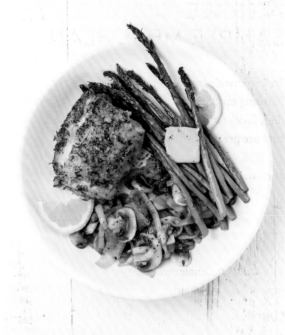

PLATE 2

- 2 cups (134 g) chopped kale
- ½ avocado
- ½ cup (75 g) chopped apple
- 2 tablespoons (15 g) chopped walnuts
- 1 tablespoon (15 ml) olive oil–based salad dressing
- ½ cup (100 g) roasted winter squash
- One 4-ounce (115 g) grass-fed steak

PLATE 3

- 8 spears roasted asparagus with avocado oil
- 1 cup (weight varies) sautéed mushrooms and onions with avocado oil
- 1 or 2 roasted chicken thighs

"EATING A DIET FULL OF WHOLE FOODS MEANS TIME MUST BE SPENT PLANNING, SHOPPING, AND PREPARING."

A THREE-DAY SAMPLE MEAL PLAN

To keep meals fun and interesting, instead of focusing on the foods that are not part of the pegan diet, focus on the many delicious, nutritious foods that are great for your body.

When shopping, I typically buy the same foods and swap seasonal produce throughout the year.

Use the 75 percent/25 percent plate model (see page 17) to create healthy meals.

DAY 1

BREAKFAST: Omelet with arugula, tomatoes, and goat cheese and a side of asparagus

LUNCH: Kale salad topped with chickpeas, diced cooked chicken, avocado, radish, and diced apple, topped with an olive oil–based salad dressing

DINNER: Roasted salmon with roasted sweet potatoes and broccoli

SNACKS OR SWEET TREATS: Raw or roasted cashews and berries with 85 percent dark chocolate

DAY 2

BREAKFAST: Breakfast salad of arugula, raspberries, pecans, and avocado topped with two poached eggs, tossed in an olive oil–based salad dressing

LUNCH: Deli turkey slices wrapped around cheese, avocado, and fermented vegetables, like sauerkraut, served with cherry tomatoes, cucumber slices, and a small handful of almonds

DINNER: Grass-fed steak with roasted Brussels sprouts and a salad of dark leafy greens with an olive oil–based salad dressing and walnuts

SNACKS OR SWEET TREATS: Olives and veggie sticks with hummus; chia seed pudding with berries

DAY 3

BREAKFAST: Lettuce wraps filled with nitrate-free bacon or sausage, eggs, tomatoes, and chopped purple cabbage; add salsa, guacamole, or sliced jalapeño peppers

LUNCH: Broth-based soup with veggies and chicken

DINNER: Pan-seared lamb chops with roasted carrots and cauliflower

SNACKS OR SWEET TREATS: ½ apple with almond butter; jicama slices topped with avocado and pumpkin seeds

MEAL PREPPING

The key to any healthy-eating lifestyle is planning. Eating a diet full of whole foods means time must be spent planning, shopping, and preparing. With a busy lifestyle, this can feel overwhelming.

TIPS FOR MEAL PREP

CREATE A SCHEDULE AND ROUTINE to plan, shop, and prep meals each week. I like to plan my meals for the week on Saturdays and shop and prep on Sundays. This means when things get busy on Monday, I have healthy options that don't take long to cook.

LEAN ON CONVENIENCE OPTIONS when necessary. I find having precut veggies on hand makes throwing a panful into the oven quick and mindless. I usually have chopped broccoli and cauliflower in my fridge ready to go. Also, many organic chicken and grass-fed beef options are available in the freezer section, like premade burger patties or sausages. These are great for quick lunches or speedy dinners.

FIND RECIPES YOU AND YOUR FAMILY ENJOY and make them on a regular basis. I like having a cabbage salad or a healthy slow cooker meal ready to go. Cabbage salads are hearty and, even when tossed in a dressing, usually last up to four days in the refrigerator. It's easy to prepare slow cooker meals by combining meats and sauce ingredients in freezer bags or glass storage containers and keeping them frozen until needed.

MAKE SALAD DRESSINGS, DIPS, OR SAUCES AHEAD to add flavor and put meals together faster. These usually don't take long to make but having them made ahead means one less thing to think about on a busy weeknight.

KEEP CHOPPED, WASHED VEGGIES ON HAND for snacks or to top salads. I like to have cherry tomatoes, cucumber slices, carrot sticks, broccoli, and snap peas ready to go.

PREPARE ROASTED NUTS to keep on hand. Be aware that many packaged roasted nuts are made with unhealthy oils. Tossing nuts with avocado oil and salt and roasting them for 12 to 15 minutes is an easy way to ensure you're snacking healthy.

INVOLVING THE FAMILY IN A PEGAN LIFESTYLE

One of the biggest challenges for families looking to clean up their diets is finding foods and recipes everyone enjoys. Kids are often picky and influenced by the foods they see other kids eat at school or when away from home.

Consistently offer whole foods to help shift your child's mind-set when it comes to clean eating. It's also important to back up your offerings with explanations. Why should they eat cashews instead of chips? Why do we have homemade almond flour cookies instead of the blue-packaged alternative from the store? Giving your child information about your dietary choices empowers them to understand your motives.

With a little effort, you will find healthier alternatives to their favorite foods, such as:

- Chicken fingers with almond flour coating
- Cookies made with almond flour and dark chocolate chips
- Homemade chicken soup with rice or millet instead of noodles
- Homemade crackers made with almond flour
- Pizza on homemade cauliflower crust

Including kids in the decision-making process also helps them buy into your new way of eating. Help your kids get involved by:

- Showing kids recipes you plan to try and asking their opinion of it. Let them browse cookbooks or Pinterest with you when looking for new recipes to feed the family.
- Taking kids grocery shopping and explaining that the healthiest foods for our bodies come from the perimeter of the store and not usually from a box or plastic bag. Model healthy food choices and let them choose fruits, vegetables, or meats they would like to try.
- Including kids in food preparation. Younger children can wash produce or stir batters. Older children can help with chopping and cooking. Getting kids in the kitchen not only helps them understand the value of cooking their own food, but it also sets them up with the skills they need to continue eating healthy into adulthood.

CHAPTER 2

BREAKFAST

Starting the day with an energizing meal sets the tone for the rest of the day. Our bodies and brains need healthy fats, protein, and fiber for optimal functioning. Conventional breakfast fare offers little in the way of nutrients. Flipping the idea of breakfast and focusing your morning meal on quality protein sources, vibrant produce, and healthy fats ensures your body has the nutrients it needs—even if the rest of the day doesn't go as planned. This chapter contains both squeaky-clean breakfast options as well as breakfast treats. Try to start most days with a meal centered on low glycemic index vegetables and quality protein sources and save the other foods for occasional treats.

COLLARD GREEN BREAKFAST WRAPS

Collard greens are an easy, nutrient-dense way to wrap up your breakfast. This breakfast burrito–style wrap is made with classic fillings and is high in both protein and fiber.

FOR PICKLED RED ONIONS:

¾ cup (180 ml) apple cider vinegar

1 tablespoon (20 g) maple syrup

1 teaspoon sea salt

1 large red onion, thinly sliced

FOR COLLARD WRAPS:

4 collard greens

1 cup (256 g) black beans

½ avocado, peeled and sliced

2 large pastured eggs, scrambled

4 bacon slices, cooked

½ cup (80 g) pickled red onions

Salsa, for dipping

To make the pickled onions: In a small saucepan over medium heat, combine the vinegar, maple syrup, and salt. Bring the mixture to a low simmer.

Place the sliced red onion in a jar or small container and pour the hot vinegar mixture over the top. Let soak for at least 1 hour, or refrigerate overnight.

To make the collard wraps: Soak the collard leaves in warm water for 20 minutes while preparing the filling ingredients.

Cut the protruding side of the collard leaf stem off the inner side of each leaf and trim off the stem at the bottom of the leaf.

Place two leaves, side by side, stem-side up, with the two stem ends overlapping each other. Into the center of the leaves, place half each of the black beans, avocado, eggs, bacon, and pickled red onions. Fold both top ends of the leaves to the center, covering the fillings. Similar to wrapping a burrito, fold one side to the center and roll up the bundle. Repeat with the remaining leaves and filling. Halve the wraps and serve with salsa for dipping.

Refrigerate leftover pickled red onions in an airtight container for up to 1 week.

YIELD

2 SERVINGS

NUTRITIONAL ANALYSIS

PER SERVING (1 BURRITO):

463 CALORIES

30G FAT

21G PROTEIN

30G CARBOHYDRATE

12G DIETARY FIBER

NOTE

If you do not soak the collard greens before use, the wraps will still taste delicious. Soaking the greens softens them so they don't tear as easily when folding

ADD IT!

Use this as a template to build your perfect breakfast wrap: Sausage, ham, or leftover chicken are all great additions for protein. Goat cheese or raw Cheddar adds a lot of flavor to these wraps. I like to use something that spreads on for the first layer, but if you don't want to use black beans, choose hummus, guacamole, or sweet potato purée.

SAVORY VEGETABLE PANCAKES

These delicious savory pancakes have a gingery bite and are a filling and fiber-rich way to start the day. Fats aid our bodies in absorbing carotenoids from vegetables, the nutrients that help our bodies ward off heart disease and cancer. Lightly pan-frying these until golden not only creates a delicious crispy exterior, but it also increases the nutrition available to our bodies. My favorite combination is cabbage, carrot, onion, and kale, but this recipe is 100 percent customizable. Use up those veggies lingering in your fridge. Shredded sweet potato, zucchini, or even cauliflower rice or chopped broccoli are great in this mix.

4 cups (280 g) shredded green cabbage, or a mix of green and red

2 cups (134 g) very thinly sliced lacinato kale

2 carrots, shredded

½ large onion, very thinly sliced

½ cup (48 g) almond flour

¼ cup (60 ml) coconut aminos

2 tablespoons (30 ml) rice wine vinegar

1 tablespoon (8 g) grated peeled fresh ginger

1 teaspoon sea salt

5 large pastured eggs, beaten

Avocado oil

In a large bowl, mix the cabbage, kale, carrots, and onion. Use your hands to toss the vegetables to combine. Add the almond flour, coconut aminos, vinegar, ginger, and salt. Use your hands again to toss and fully coat all the vegetables. Be sure to break up the ginger so it is evenly spread throughout the veggie mixture.

Stir in the beaten eggs and evenly coat the veggies with them.

Heat a large skillet over medium-low heat and add enough oil for frying (2 to 3 tablespoons, or 30 to 45 ml).

Working in batches, scoop ½ cup (about 120 g) of the vegetable mixture, compress it in a measuring cup used to scoop out a portion, then turn it out into the hot skillet. Cook for about 10 minutes, pressing the fritter down with a spatula occasionally. Flip and cook the other side for 6 to 8 minutes, or until both sides are lightly golden brown. Repeat with the remaining vegetable mixture until all fritters are cooked. Serve hot.

YIELD

4 SERVINGS (8 PANCAKES)

NUTRITIONAL ANALYSIS

PER SERVING (2 PANCAKES):

173 CALORIES

13G FAT

6G PROTEIN

9G CARBOHYDRATE

3G DIETARY FIBER

NOTE

Avocado oil is ideal for frying savory dishes. Its high smoke point means the fats aren't damaged during cooking at high temperatures. The nutrients and phytochemicals in oils with lower smoke points, like extra-virgin olive oil, are destroyed when heated past their smoke point.

ADD IT!

To substitute other veggies you have on hand, keep the overall quantities similar. For example, use 2 cups (140 g) shredded cabbage and 2 cups (140 g) shredded zucchini or sweet potato instead of the 4 cups (280 g) cabbage.

BUCKWHEAT PANCAKES WITH BLUEBERRY SYRUP

Buckwheat groats are not actually grains. They are considered a "pseudo cereal," being actually a seed. Although grains are limited on a pegan diet, buckwheat is recommended in moderation because it is gluten-free, is rich in minerals, and contains high-quality proteins. These fluffy, protein-packed pancakes are made in a blender and are lightly sweetened by the fruit. Take your breakfast up a notch with blueberry maple syrup.

FOR BLUEBERRY SYRUP:

1 cup (155 g) frozen blueberries

2 tablespoons (30 ml) water

2 tablespoons (40 g) maple syrup

1 tablespoon (12 g) chia seeds

FOR PANCAKES:

6 tablespoons (45 g) raw buckwheat groats

3 large pastured eggs

1 banana

½ teaspoon baking powder

¼ teaspoon sea salt

¼ teaspoon ground cinnamon

¼ cup (24 g) almond flour

Coconut oil cooking spray, for cooking

To make the blueberry syrup: In a small saucepan over medium heat, combine the blueberries, water, and maple syrup. Bring to a simmer. Once the mixture reaches a simmer, gently smash the berries with a spoon and cook for about 5 minutes more. Remove the syrup from the heat.

Sprinkle the chia seeds over the top. Stir to incorporate and let sit for about 10 minutes to thicken before serving.

To make the pancakes: In a blender, process the buckwheat groats into a fine flour. Set aside.

In the blender, combine the eggs, banana, baking powder, salt, and cinnamon. Process the mixture until smooth and creamy.

Add 6 tablespoons (48 g) of buckwheat flour (you should have just enough) and the almond flour. Pulse several times until the flours are incorporated.

YIELD

6 PANCAKES

NUTRITIONAL ANALYSIS

PER SERVING (1 PANCAKE, 2 TABLESPOONS, OR 30 ML, SYRUP):

167 CALORIES

6G FAT

6G PROTEIN

25G CARBOHYDRATE

4G DIETARY FIBER

NOTE

The syrup is equally delicious made with other berries. Try strawberries, raspberries, or blackberries. I've also used chopped peaches for a similar fruit topping.

ADD IT!

Experiment with your favorite pancake add-ins. Blueberries, strawberries, and banana slices are a great way to change up these pancakes.

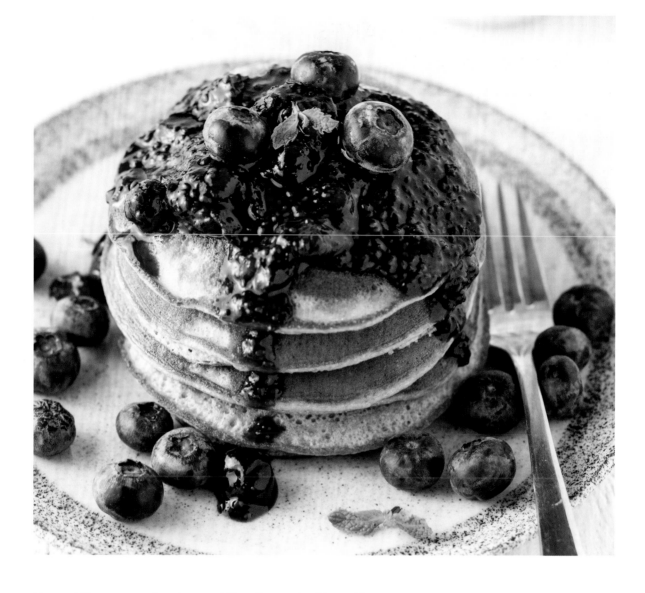

Heat a skillet over medium heat and liberally coat it with cooking spray.

In ¼-cup (60 ml) portions, pour the batter into the hot skillet. The batter will seem thin, but it cooks into light, fluffy, thick pancakes. Cook the pancakes slowly until air bubbles start to form on the tops, 3 to 5 minutes. Flip the pancakes and cook the other side until they are lightly golden brown, 3 to 5 minutes more.

NOTE

Store-bought buckwheat flour is made from toasted buck-wheat, which has a strong flavor. Using raw buckwheat groats, which are light brown and green in color, yields better-tasting baked goods.

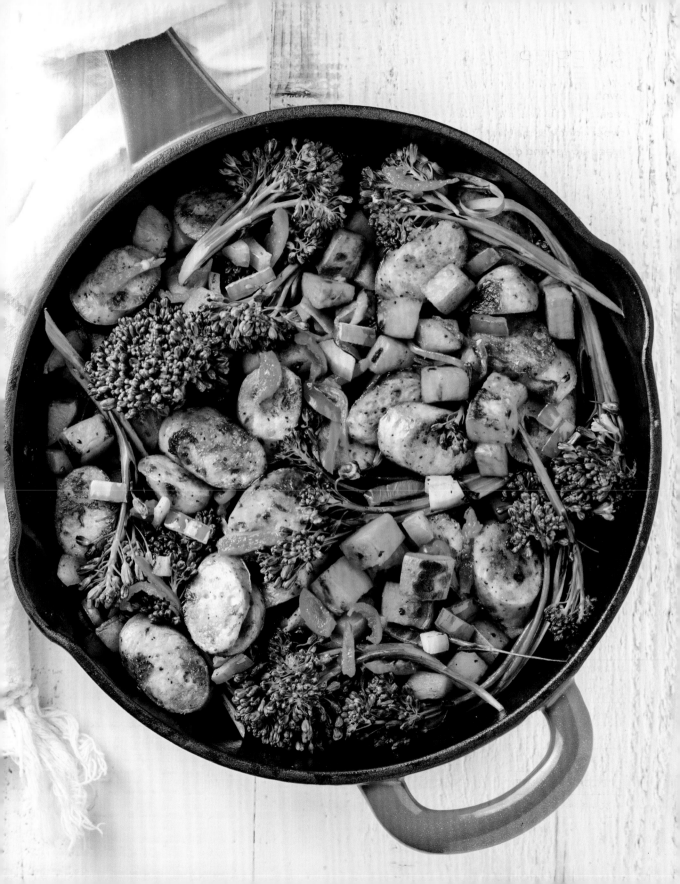

SWEET POTATO SKILLET

Sweet potatoes are higher on the glycemic index, so save meals like this for days requiring extra energy. This hearty, nutritious meal comes together quickly if the sweet potatoes are chopped ahead. Broccolini, or even broccoli rabe, adds some green power and a fresh taste to this filling breakfast skillet.

3 tablespoons (45 ml) avocado oil

2 medium-size sweet potatoes, diced

Sea salt and black pepper to taste

½ cup (80 g) diced red onion

12 ounces (340 g) precooked organic chicken sausage links, sliced

One 3-ounce (85 g) bunch broccolini, trimmed

3 peppadew peppers, sliced (optional)

In a large skillet over medium-low heat, combine the oil and sweet potatoes. Season with salt and pepper to taste. Sauté the potatoes for 12 to 15 minutes until soft, stirring every couple of minutes for even browning.

When the potatoes are soft, add the red onion and cook, stirring, for 8 to 10 minutes more until the onion is softened.

Add the sliced sausage and broccolini to the skillet and stir to mix into the sweet potatoes. Cover the skillet and let the sausage and broccolini heat through for about 8 minutes.

Taste and season with more salt and pepper, if necessary, and garnish with peppadew peppers (if using). Serve hot.

YIELD

4 SERVINGS

NUTRITIONAL ANALYSIS

PER SERVING (1½ CUPS):

328 CALORIES

21G FAT

17G PROTEIN

17G CARBOHYDRATE

3G DIETARY FIBER

NOTE

Peppadew peppers are spicy, sweet pickled peppers. Using them as a garnish adds a tangy contrast to the sweet potatoes. They can be difficult to find. Look for them at the olive bar in your local grocery, pick up a jar at a gourmet grocer, substitute another pickled pepper, or omit them.

ADD IT!

This skillet is a great template for lots of different breakfast options. Keep the sweet potatoes and sausage but use any other veggies you like in a stir-fry in place of the broccolini. Zucchini, chopped kale, and bell pepper are great additions.

LEMON-RASPBERRY BUCKWHEAT MUFFINS

Buckwheat is low on the glycemic index, a key consideration when choosing foods on the pegan diet. Its nutrients are slowly absorbed by the body, making baked goods made with buckwheat more filling and energizing. These muffins are made with a combination of buckwheat flour and almond flour, giving you a higher protein option than the standard bakery fare.

FOR STREUSEL TOPPING:

¼ cup (23 g) sliced almonds

2 tablespoons (15 g) buckwheat flour

2 tablespoons (20 g) coconut sugar

2 tablespoons (28 g) pastured butter, melted

FOR MUFFINS

1 cup (120 g) raw buckwheat groats

1 cup (96 g) almond flour

6 tablespoons (54 g) coconut sugar

2 teaspoons baking powder

1 teaspoon sea salt

2 small ripe bananas

4 large pastured eggs

½ cup (1 stick; 112 g) pastured butter, melted

2 teaspoons vanilla extract

3 tablespoons (18 g) grated lemon zest

3 tablespoons (45 ml) fresh lemon juice

1½ cups (190 g) organic raspberries, fresh or frozen

To make the streusel topping: In a small bowl, stir together the streusel topping ingredients. Set aside.

To make the muffins: In a blender, process the buckwheat groats until a light, fine flour forms. Measure and reserve 1 cup (100 g) of buckwheat flour for this recipe and store any remaining flour in an airtight container for future use.

Preheat the oven to 350°F (180°C, or gas mark 4). Prepare a standard muffin tin by lining it with parchment paper liners. Using parchment liners rather than standard cupcake papers ensures the muffins slip out easily. Set aside.

In a large bowl, whisk the reserved buckwheat flour, almond flour, coconut sugar, baking powder, and salt to mix the dry ingredients fully.

In a medium-size bowl, mash the bananas with a fork into a purée. Add the eggs, melted butter, vanilla, lemon zest, and lemon juice. Mix well. Pour the wet ingredients into the dry ingredients, and stir to combine, using fewer than 10 strokes.

Fold the raspberries into the batter. Evenly divide the batter among the 12 liners. Top each muffin with 1 heaping teaspoon of streusel topping.

Bake for 25 to 28 minutes until the centers are set.

Let cool completely. Refrigerate leftovers in an airtight container for up to 7 days, or freeze for up to 3 months.

NOTE

Gluten-free flours dry out faster than wheat flour, so do not overbake these muffins.

YIELD

12 MUFFINS

NUTRITIONAL ANALYSIS

PER SERVING (1 MUFFIN):

270 CALORIES

17G FAT

6G PROTEIN

26G CARBOHYDRATE

4G DIETARY FIBER

NOTE

Raw buckwheat groats are light brown and green in color and are often found in the bulk section of health food stores. Pre-ground buckwheat flour is toasted, and the flavor is stronger than raw buckwheat.

ADD IT!

These muffins are a great canvas for lots of muffin recipes. Rather than the raspberries, add sliced strawberries or blueberries. These would also be great with dark chocolate chips. Experiment by adding ⅓ cup (40 g) chopped walnuts or (37 g) pecans, or use either one as a substitution for the almonds in the streusel topping.

SAUSAGE, ZUCCHINI, AND APPLE FRITTERS

Mix up your breakfast routine with these veggie and sausage fritters. Sausage provides a great protein boost and the apple adds a sweet-tart bite. For the healthiest option, purchase organic sausage sweetened only with maple syrup, not refined sugar. Feel free to be heavy-handed with the black pepper—a great contrast to the sweet flavors. I like these fritters served over a bed of arugula with a few slices of avocado.

4 cups (480 g) grated zucchini

1½ cups (225 g) diced apple
(I like Pink Lady or Honeycrisp)

1 tablespoon (3 g) chopped
fresh sage

½ teaspoon sea salt

Black pepper to taste

12 ounces (340 g) organic maple
breakfast sausage

1 large pastured egg

3 tablespoons (45 ml) avocado oil

In a large bowl, combine the zucchini, apple, sage, salt, and pepper to taste. Use a fork to mix the ingredients well.

Add the sausage and egg and mix with a fork to combine with the other ingredients. The sausage might be sticky and difficult to incorporate, but continue gently pressing and spreading it into the zucchini mixture.

Heat a skillet over medium-low heat and drizzle in the avocado oil.

Working in batches, scoop ¼ cup (about 80 g) of the mixture, compact it into a patty, and add it to the hot skillet. Use a spatula to flatten each mound slightly. Cover the skillet and cook for about 10 minutes. Flip each fritter, leaving skillet uncovered, and cook for 6 to 8 minutes more to brown the other side. Repeat with the remaining zucchini mixture until all the fritters are cooked. Serve hot.

Cool any leftovers and refrigerate them in an airtight container for up to 3 days.

YIELD

14 FRITTERS

NUTRITIONAL ANALYSIS

PER SERVING (1 FRITTER):

148 CALORIES

12G FAT

6G PROTEIN

5G CARBOHYDRATE

2G DIETARY FIBER

NOTE

The apple in these fritters adds great flavor, but use another shredded veggie in place of it, if you prefer. Try shredded carrot or cauliflower rice.

ENDURANCE CHIA SEED PUDDING WITH BERRIES

Swap your oatmeal for this delicious easy-to-make chia seed pudding. The Tarahumara Peoples of Mexico run 50 to 100 miles at a time and credit their incredible endurance to these powerful seeds. Chia seeds are rich in omega-3, protein, and calcium and absolutely burst with fiber. The seeds absorb ten times their weight in water and thicken liquid to a puddinglike texture similar to tapioca. I prefer making chia pudding with almond milk rather than coconut milk because it lasts longer in the fridge (coconut milk sours after 2 to 3 days).

3 cups (720 ml) unsweetened vanilla Almond Milk (page 173) or store-bought almond milk

2 to 3 tablespoons (40 to 60 g) maple syrup or honey

2 tablespoons (28 g) virgin coconut oil, melted

½ cup (96 g) chia seeds

¼ teaspoon vanilla extract or almond extract

Fresh berries, such as blackberries, blueberries, raspberries, or strawberries, for topping (optional)

Unsweetened shredded coconut, for topping (optional)

Chopped nuts or seeds, for topping (optional)

Nut butter, for topping (optional)

Chopped 85% dark chocolate, for topping (optional)

In a blender, combine the almond milk and maple syrup. Blend on low speed. While the blender is running, add the melted coconut oil and process until incorporated.

Add the chia seeds and vanilla and pulse to combine. Let sit for 5 to 10 minutes, then pulse 4 or 5 times. Repeat 3 or 4 times until the pudding is thickened.

Pour the pudding into storage jars. I like to use small jars, so they are easy to take with me on the go or pull out and top for a quick breakfast or snack. The pudding will continue to thicken as it chills, so it's best to make it several hours before serving. Top as desired when ready to serve.

The chia seed pudding will keep for 5 to 6 days, refrigerated in airtight jars.

(continued)

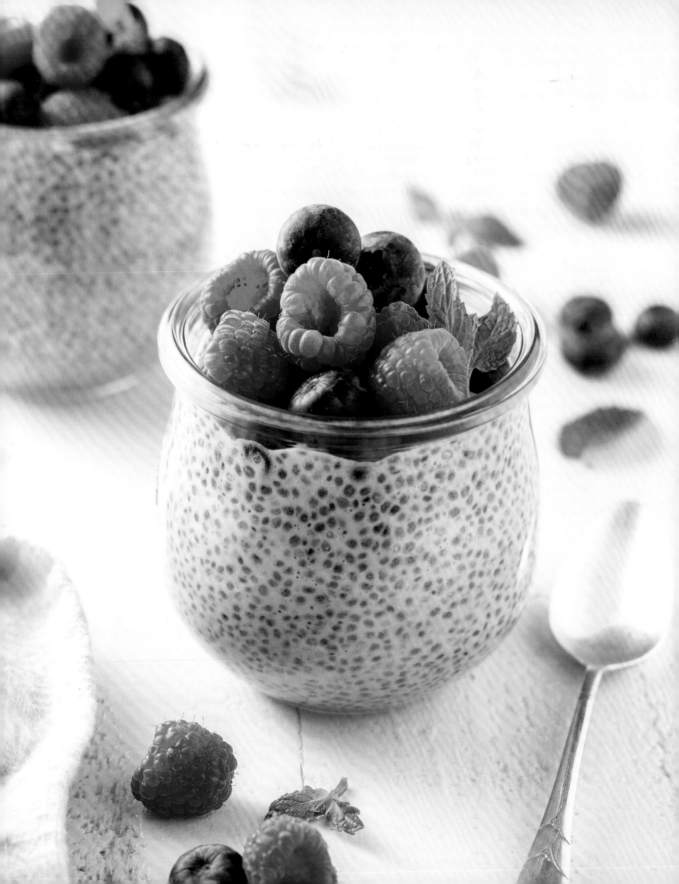

8 SERVINGS

NUTRITIONAL ANALYSIS

PER SERVING (½ CUP, 103 G, PUDDING WITH NO TOPPINGS):

173 CALORIES

13G FAT

4G PROTEIN

13G CARBOHYDRATE

6G DIETARY FIBER

NOTE

The absorbency of chia seeds varies depending on the age of the seeds and the brand. If the pudding seems too thin, add another 2 to 3 tablespoons (24 to 36 g) of chia seeds. If it's too thick, add another 2 to 3 tablespoons (30 to 45 ml) of almond milk. You can also make this pudding sugar-free by substituting monk fruit sweetener or stevia to taste.

ADD IT!

This basic recipe is adaptable. Add ¼ cup (22 g) cocoa powder plus an extra 1 to 2 tablespoons (20 to 40 g) of maple syrup for a chocolate option. It's also delicious with ½ cup (85 g) chopped strawberries or (65 g) raspberries blended into the almond milk, similar to a flavored yogurt.

POWER-UP MILLET BREAKFAST BOWL

Power-up your day with high-protein millet breakfast bowls. Millet provides sustained energy, fiber, and an extra boost of protein. I love savory millet bowls topped with eggs and sautéed veggies. These bowls would be equally delicious topped with bacon, sautéed kale, zucchini, or bell peppers. A sprinkling of goat cheese makes them extra special.

2 tablespoons (30 ml) avocado oil, divided

2 cups (140 g) sliced mushrooms

2 cups (298 g) cherry tomatoes

Sea salt and black pepper to taste

1 cup (200 g) millet, cooked according to the package directions

4 cups (80 g) arugula

4 large pastured eggs, cooked to your liking

¼ cup (38 g) goat cheese crumbles

In a large skillet over medium heat, heat 1 tablespoon (15 ml) of the avocado oil. Add the mushrooms and tomatoes. Sauté for 5 to 7 minutes until the tomatoes burst and the mushrooms have started to brown. Set aside.

Drizzle the remaining 1 tablespoon (15 ml) of avocado oil into the hot millet, then season it with salt and pepper to taste. Evenly divide the millet among 4 bowls.

Top each bowl with one-fourth of the sautéed mushrooms and tomatoes, 1 cup (20 g) of arugula, and 1 egg. Sprinkle each with 1 tablespoon (about 9 g) of goat cheese.

YIELD

4 SERVINGS

NUTRITIONAL ANALYSIS

PER SERVING (½ CUP, OR 87 G, COOKED MILLET, 1 EGG, AND TOPPINGS):

380 CALORIES

17G FAT

16G PROTEIN

42G CARBOHYDRATE

6G DIETARY FIBER

NOTE

Millet is cooked with a ratio of 2 cups (480 ml) water per 1 cup (200 g) grain. Let sit, covered, for 10 minutes after cooking, then fluff the millet with a fork. Millet is best the day it's cooked fresh, but if you need to reheat leftovers, add a few tablespoons (about 45 ml) of water or chicken broth and reheat it covered.

ADD IT!

Make these bowls with whatever ingredients you have on hand. Sauté any veggies you have in your crisper and swap the eggs for bacon, sausage, or even leftover cooked beef or chicken. I also love these bowls with a spoonful of homemade pesto on top.

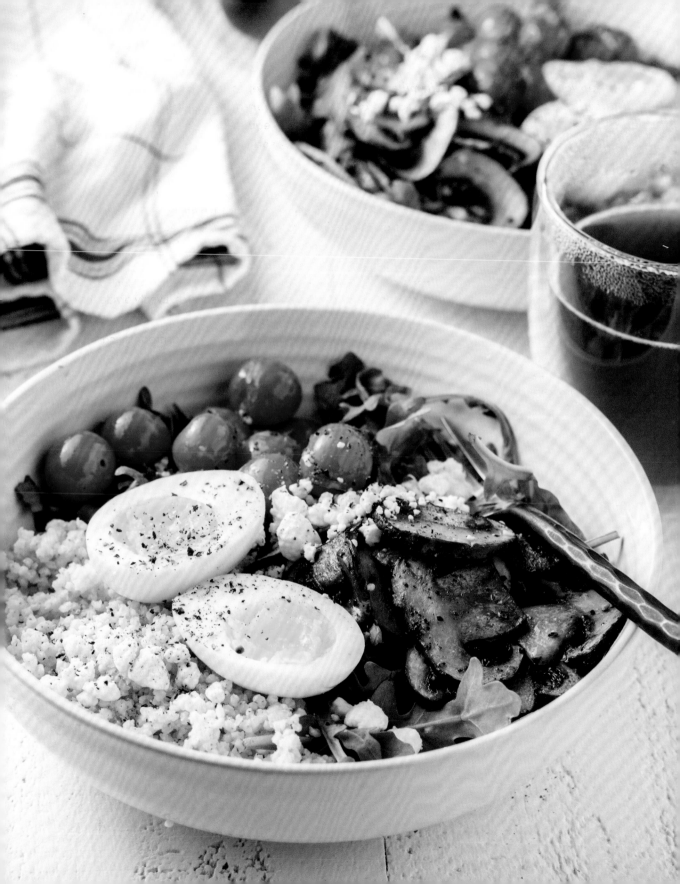

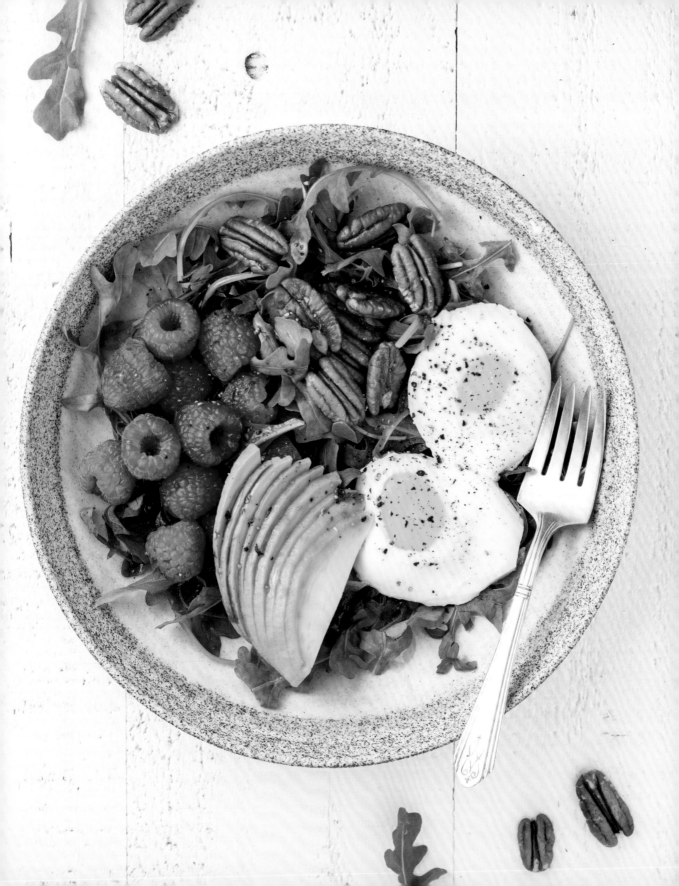

BREAKFAST ARUGULA SALAD

Start your day by checking off a big serving of greens. This breakfast salad, or a variation of it, is my go-to breakfast because it's filling, and if my day gets out of hand, I know I started it with everything my body needs. Breakfast salads are great with a variety of greens—from spinach to kale or arugula. Arugula is my favorite because it stays fresh all week long and has a pleasant peppery bite, which is tasty with the creamy avocado and sweet pecans. Throw in any kind of berries you have or add bacon if you need more protein. If you need a grab-and-go option, kale makes a great make-ahead breakfast salad because it won't wilt as it sits dressed and topped in the fridge.

2 cups (40 g) arugula

½ cup (63 g) fresh raspberries

2 tablespoons (14 g) pecans

¼ avocado, peeled and cut into chunks

1 tablespoon Balsamic Dijon Vinaigrette (page 148) or Easy Lemon Vinaigrette (page 148)

2 large pastured eggs, cooked to your liking

On a plate, arrange the arugula, raspberries, pecans, and avocado. Drizzle with the vinaigrette. Top the salad with the cooked eggs.

YIELD

1 SERVING

NUTRITIONAL ANALYSIS

PER SERVING:

380 CALORIES

32G FAT

16G PROTEIN

10G CARBOHYDRATE

5G DIETARY FIBER

NOTE

Fat helps the body absorb nutrients, so pairing greens with an olive oil–based dressing and other healthy fatty foods, like eggs, nuts, and avocado, ensures the best absorption.

ADD IT!

Experiment with your favorite greens, berries, nuts, or seeds.

SHEET PAN BUTTERNUT SQUASH HASH

This sheet pan breakfast is a great weekend meal when you have a little more time to cook. Cubes of squash, along with bell pepper, onion, and spices, are roasted until sweet, then made into "nests" with baked eggs. Sprinkle with goat cheese, or try topped with your favorite salsa and avocado slices. If you don't have a crowd to feed, the hash keeps well and is great reheated.

1 butternut squash, peeled, halved, seeded, and cubed

½ red bell pepper, diced

½ green bell pepper, diced

½ yellow onion, diced

2 tablespoons (30 ml) avocado oil

2 teaspoons sea salt, plus more for seasoning

1 tablespoon (7 g) ground cumin

1 tablespoon (8 g) chili powder

¼ teaspoon cayenne pepper

Black pepper to taste

8 large pastured eggs

Goat cheese crumbles, for garnish (optional)

Preheat the oven to 425°F (220°C, or gas mark 7).

On a large sheet pan, combine the butternut squash, red and green bell peppers, and onion. Drizzle the vegetables with the oil and season with the salt, cumin, chili powder, cayenne, and black pepper to taste. Use your hands to toss the veggies, evenly coating them in the oil and seasonings.

Bake the hash for 30 minutes. Remove from the oven. Use a spatula to divide the hash into 8 equal mounds, and make an indentation in the center of each. Crack 1 egg into the center of each mound. Season with more salt and pepper to taste.

Return the sheet pan to the oven and bake for 10 to 15 minutes more, depending on your desired doneness for the eggs.

Sprinkle the hash with goat cheese (if using) to serve.

YIELD

4 SERVINGS

NUTRITIONAL ANALYSIS

PER SERVING (1 CUP, OR 200 G, VEGGIES PLUS 2 EGGS):

300 CALORIES

16G FAT

15G PROTEIN

28G CARBOHYDRATE

5G DIETARY FIBER

NOTE

Chopping the butternut squash into small cubes helps when forming the hash into nests to cook the eggs in. You can save time buying pre-chopped butternut squash. Another time-saving tip is not to peel the squash. The peel softens when baked and adds fiber to the dish.

ADD IT!

This hash is great with bacon added. Cook the bacon, then crumble it and mix it into the hash when adding the eggs.

CHAPTER 3

◆ ◆ ◆

SIMPLE SNACKS

Prepping healthy and energizing snacks is the best way to stay on track throughout the day. Fresh foods are always best, so keeping chopped veggies and fresh fruit on hand is a great place to start. Try adding some of these nut, seed, and veggie-based recipes to your rotation to mix things up and keep your diet interesting. These simple ideas are sure to become family favorites.

GARLIC AND ROSEMARY ALMOND MEAL FLAXSEED CRACKERS

These crunchy, savory crackers are perfect for loading up with your favorite toppings. Serve with soup, use as salad croutons, or enjoy as a snack on their own. I love adding garlic and rosemary for a delicious layer of flavor, but omit the savory seasonings and use the crackers as a vessel for nut butter and fruit.

(pictured on page 47)

1½ cups (218 g) raw almonds

¼ cup (42 g) flaxseed

2 tablespoons (3 g) finely chopped fresh rosemary leaves

½ teaspoon sea salt

1 or 2 garlic cloves, peeled

¼ cup (60 ml) water

Preheat the oven to 325°F (170°C, or gas mark 3).

In a blender, combine the almonds and flaxseed. Process until a flour forms. Do not overprocess or the nuts will start to become nut butter. Transfer to a medium-size bowl.

Add the rosemary and salt. Using a Microplane, grate the garlic into the bowl. Stir to combine the ingredients evenly.

Add the water and stir to form a ball of dough. Place the dough ball on a sheet of parchment paper and top it with another sheet of parchment. Use a rolling pin to spread the dough into a rectangle about 10 × 12 inches (25 × 30 cm). Gently peel off the top layer of parchment. Use a pizza cutter to cut the dough into 1-inch (2.5 cm) squares. Slide the parchment with the crackers onto a baking sheet.

Bake the crackers for 22 to 26 minutes until the edges are golden brown. Turn off the oven and let some heat escape. Leave the baking sheet in the oven with the door ajar for at least 10 minutes more so the crackers fully crisp.

YIELD

10 SERVINGS

NUTRITIONAL ANALYSIS

PER SERVING (12 CRACKERS):

117 CALORIES

10G FAT

4G PROTEIN

5G CARBOHYDRATE

3G DIETARY FIBER

NOTE

Make these crackers more kid friendly by using 1¾ cups (168 g) blanched almond flour rather than whole almonds and flaxseed, producing crackers that look more like a store-bought option.

ADD IT!

If you don't have flaxseed, try hemp, chia, or sesame seeds instead.

CHIA SEED POWER CRACKERS

These deliciously crunchy crackers are packed with nutrients thanks to lots of seeds. They make a delicious snack, but also a great topper for salads and soups. Add to a cheese platter with some berries for a nourishing party appetizer. I like to leave these seasoned only with salt, but add some grated fresh garlic or chopped fresh herbs if you'd like more flavor.

(pictured on page 47)

½ cup (96 g) chia seeds

½ cup (73 g) sunflower seeds

½ cup (70 g) pumpkin seeds

½ cup (72 g) sesame seeds

¼ cup (28 g) hemp seeds

¾ teaspoon sea salt

1 cup (240 ml) warm water

Preheat the oven to 300°F (150°C, or gas mark 2). Line 2 large baking sheets with parchment paper or silicone baking mats.

In a medium-size bowl, stir together all the seeds and salt. Stir in the warm water. Let sit for about 5 minutes so the chia seeds begin to absorb the liquid.

Once there is no water sitting in the bowl, transfer half the mixture to one of the prepared baking sheets. Cover the seed "dough" with a piece of parchment and use a rolling pin to flatten the dough into a large rectangle. I prefer these crackers rolled thinly, into about a 10 × 12-inch (25 × 30 cm) rectangle. Repeat with the remaining dough on the second baking sheet.

Bake one sheet at a time. Bake for 35 minutes. Gently flip the crackers over and bake for 25 minutes more until dried and firm. The crackers will crisp as they cool.

Turn off the oven and let some heat escape. Leave the baking sheet in the oven with the door ajar for at least 10 more minutes, or until the oven has fully cooled, to create the crispest crackers. Break the cooled crackers into smaller pieces to serve.

YIELD

12 SERVINGS

NUTRITIONAL ANALYSIS

PER SERVING:

170 CALORIES

14G FAT

7G PROTEIN

7G CARBOHYDRATE

5G DIETARY FIBER

NOTE

Chia seeds are known as a power food and are commonly eaten by endurance athletes. Rich in omega-3s, protein, iron, calcium, vitamins, and antioxidants, they are believed to aid in muscle recovery.

ADD IT!

This simple seed cracker recipe can be mixed up with other nuts and seeds. The chia seeds are a mandatory ingredient, as they absorb the water and gel up to hold the crackers together. Add chopped pecans, hazelnuts, or almonds for a delicious twist.

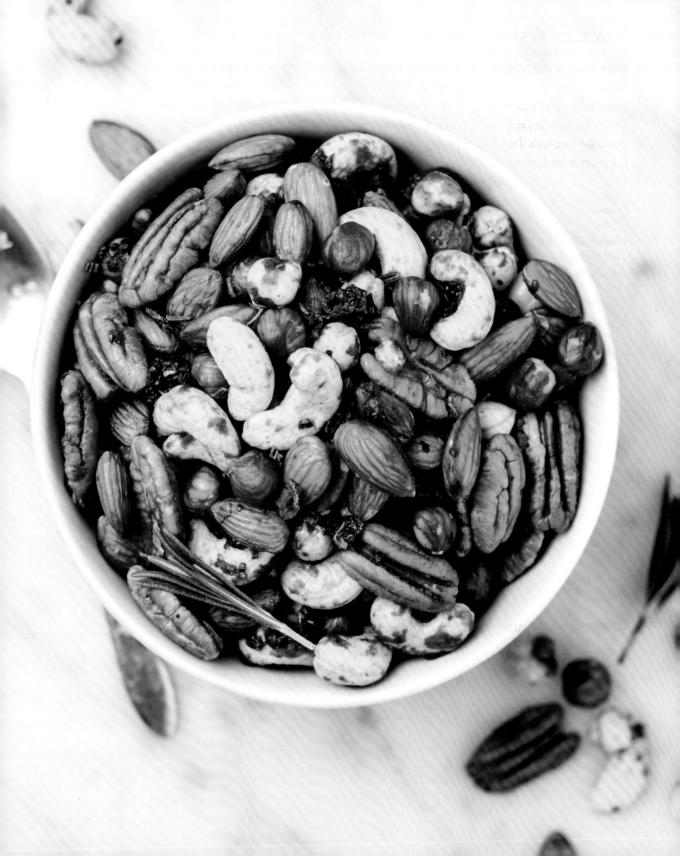

SWEET AND SPICY MIXED NUTS

Nuts are a nutritious and filling snack that provides a variety of nutrients, including magnesium and vitamin E. Because nuts are high in fat, protein, and fiber, they offer sustained energy throughout the day and minimize hunger. This delicious mix has a sweet and spicy coating and makes a great alternative to chips or crackers. I serve these as a party appetizer and keep some in the freezer for a grab-and-go snack option to tide me over until mealtime.

2 tablespoons (28 g) pastured butter

2 tablespoons (20 g) finely chopped shallot

4 cups (580 g) mixed nuts (almonds, Brazil nuts, hazelnuts, pecans, or walnuts)

2 tablespoons (3 g) finely chopped fresh rosemary leaves

2 tablespoons (18 g) coconut sugar

½ teaspoon sea salt

⅛ teaspoon cayenne pepper

Heat a skillet over medium-low heat and add the butter to melt. Add the shallot and sauté for about 10 minutes until translucent and fragrant.

Stir in the nuts. Cook for about 10 minutes, stirring occasionally to prevent burning, to toast the nuts.

Add the rosemary, coconut sugar, salt, and cayenne. Stir to coat and let the sugar melt and stick to the nuts. Once the sugar melts, remove from the heat and let the nuts cool in the skillet, stirring the mixture once or twice as it cools.

Store the nuts in an airtight container at room temperature for up to 2 days, or refrigerate for up to 1 week. If you'd like these to last longer, freeze in an airtight container for up to 3 months.

YIELD

16 SERVINGS

NUTRITIONAL ANALYSIS

PER SERVING (¼ CUP, OR ABOUT 40 G):

233 CALORIES

20G FAT

6G PROTEIN

11G CARBOHYDRATE

3G DIETARY FIBER

NOTE

These nuts make delicious holiday gifts. Fill jars with this nut blend and add a ribbon. Because of the fresh ingredients, they should be refrigerated until ready to give away. However, they will be fine for a couple of days if left under a Christmas tree.

CHICKPEA SALAD AVOCADO BOATS

*Instead of avocado toast, use avocado as the base for a delicious filling.
Avocados are rich in fiber and heart-healthy monounsaturated fatty acids,
so they satisfy hunger and keep you full for hours. These avocado boats are
filled with a tangy chickpea salad for maximum flavor.*

½ cup (120 g) canned chickpeas,
   rinsed and drained

¼ cup (37 g) quartered
   cherry tomatoes

1 tablespoon (10 g) chopped
   red onion

1½ teaspoons olive oil

1½ teaspoons fresh lemon juice

1½ teaspoons red wine vinegar

Sea salt and black pepper to taste

1 avocado, halved and pitted

In a small bowl, stir together the chickpeas, tomatoes, red onion, oil, lemon juice, and vinegar. Season with salt and pepper to taste. Fill the avocado halves with the chickpea salad and enjoy with a spoon.

YIELD

2 SERVINGS

NUTRITIONAL ANALYSIS

PER SERVING (½ AVOCADO
AND ½ CUP, ABOUT 85 G,
CHICKPEA SALAD):

266 CALORIES

18G FAT

6G PROTEIN

21G CARBOHYDRATE

10G DIETARY FIBER

NOTE

Use this avocado boat recipe as a base for whatever fillings you love. Add a chunky salsa, or an egg salad, for an equally delicious and heart-healthy snack.

SOUTHWEST ZUCCHINI CHIPS

Preparing fresh chips from vegetables other than potatoes lowers their carb content and increases the nutrient density. These zucchini chips provide a satisfying crunch and the flavor options are endless. They do take a while to bake but are quick to prep. I love these dipped in Spicy Avocado-Cilantro Dressing (page 149).

½ teaspoon onion powder

½ teaspoon garlic powder

¼ teaspoon chili powder

¼ teaspoon ground cumin

¼ teaspoon sea salt

Pinch cayenne pepper

2 large-in-diameter zucchini

1 tablespoon (15 ml) olive oil, divided

Preheat the oven to 225°F (107°C). Line 2 large baking sheets with parchment paper or silicone baking mats. Set aside.

In a small bowl, stir together the spices, salt, and cayenne. Set aside.

Use a mandoline or very sharp knife to cut the zucchini evenly into very thin chips. Arrange one-fourth of the zucchini slices on each prepared baking sheet in a single layer, being careful not to overlap them, which will cause them to steam rather than crisp while baking. Set aside the remaining chips for the next batch.

Lightly spray or brush about 1½ teaspoons of the oil onto the zucchini chips. Do not use too much oil. Sprinkle the chips with half the spice mixture, reserving the remaining oil and spice mixture for the next batch.

Place both baking sheets in the oven. Bake the zucchini for 1½ to 2 hours, switching the top and bottom sheets once about halfway through the baking time. There is no need to flip the zucchini chips. After 1½ hours, watch the zucchini and pull the chips out when they're browning, before burning, which can happen quickly.

Repeat with the remaining zucchini.

Enjoy the zucchini chips fresh, or store in an airtight container at room temperature for up to 3 days.

YIELD

4 CUPS (920 G) ZUCCHINI CHIPS

NUTRITIONAL ANALYSIS

PER SERVING (1 CUP, OR 230 G):

28 CALORIES

1G FAT

2G PROTEIN

5G CARBOHYDRATE

2G DIETARY FIBER

NOTE

Zucchini is mostly water, so these chips shrink a lot during the baking and dehydrating process. Be careful not to over season the chips. Lightly sprinkle on the seasoning. You can always add more salt later.

MEAL PREP PEGAN SNACK BOXES

One of the best ways to keep on track with any healthy eating goal is to be prepared. These meal prep snack boxes are a general idea of what you can keep on hand for grab-and-go options. Load them with your favorite veggies along with some homemade Garlic and Rosemary Almond Meal Flaxseed Crackers or Chia Seed Power Crackers and add some healthy fats such as olives or a dip.

4 servings Chia Seed Power Crackers (page 41) or Rosemary Garlic Almond Meal Flaxseed Crackers (page 40)

2 cups (238 g) cucumber slices

2 cups (298 g) cherry tomatoes

20 pitted olives

Coconut Ranch Dressing (page 153) or other dip or dressing of choice, for serving (optional)

In each of 4 airtight containers, place 1 serving of crackers, ½ cup (60 g) each of cucumber slices and (75 g) tomatoes, and 5 olives.

If desired, include a dressing or dip to serve with the boxes.

NOTE

If you don't have time to make crackers, add a mix of nuts and seeds.

ADD IT!

Instead of olives, try avocado slices or goat cheese as a healthy fat to add to these snack boxes.

YIELD

4 SNACK BOXES

NUTRITIONAL ANALYSIS

PER SERVING: VARIES

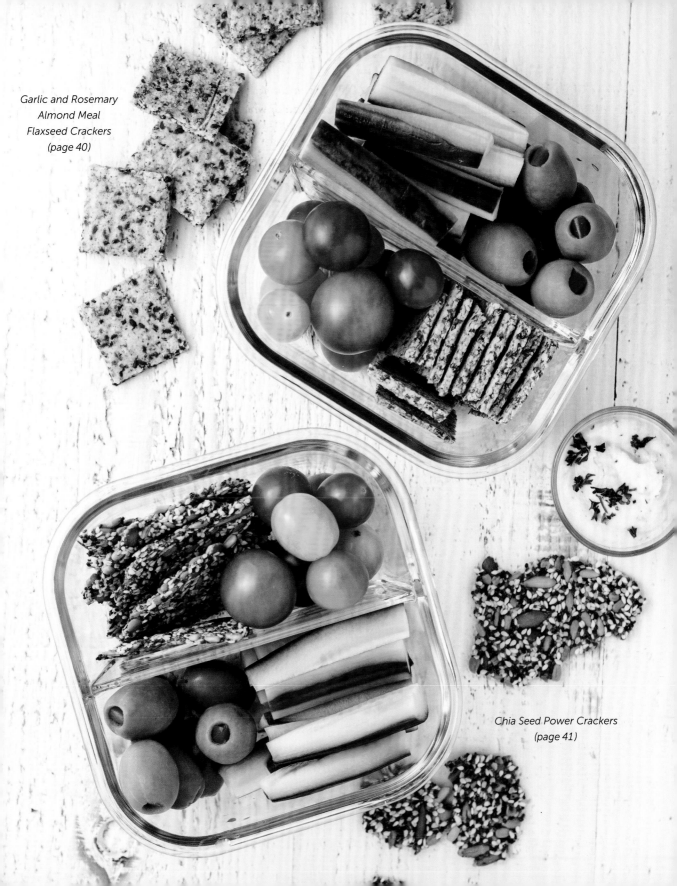

Garlic and Rosemary Almond Meal Flaxseed Crackers (page 40)

Chia Seed Power Crackers (page 41)

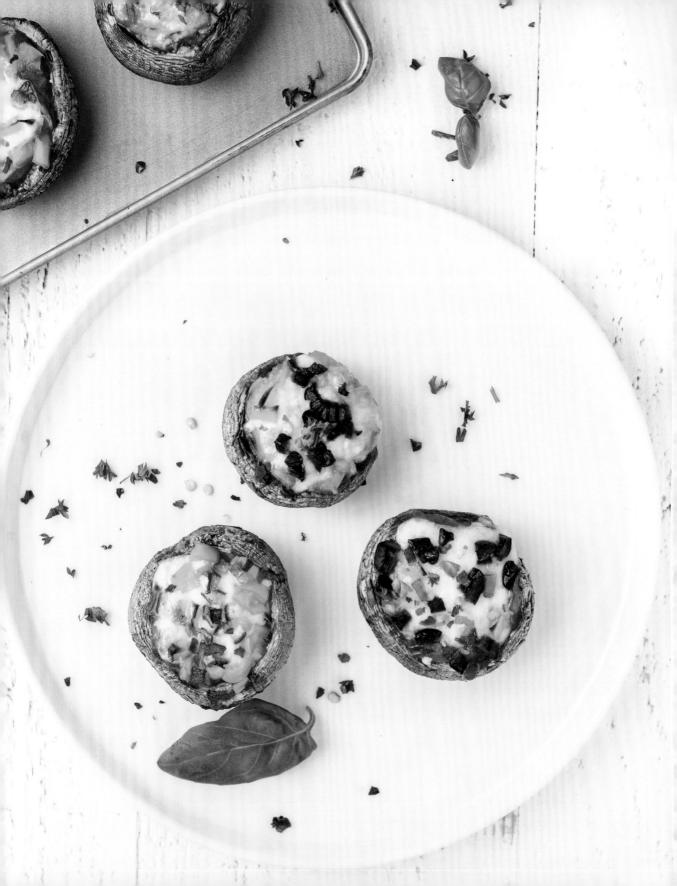

BABY PORTOBELLO PIZZA BITES

A great mini meal or snack any day, these pizza bites are made on baby portobello mushrooms, meaning they are ready to go when you are. Add your favorite pizza toppings (I love the combo used here: bell pepper, onion, and olive) and an easy-to-digest cheese, such as a raw Cheddar or goat's milk cheese.

12 baby portobello mushrooms

6 tablespoons (90 g) jarred pizza sauce

2 ounces (56 g) raw Cheddar cheese, thinly sliced

¼ bell pepper, any color, finely chopped

1 tablespoon (10 g) finely chopped red onion

5 olives, pitted and finely chopped

Preheat the oven to 425°F (220°C, or gas mark 7).

Remove the stems from the mushrooms and wash the mushrooms well. Place the mushrooms on a baking sheet, top-side down.

Fill the holes left from the stems with pizza sauce, about 1½ teaspoons per mushroom.

Top each mushroom with a thin slice of cheese and a sprinkling of bell pepper, red onion, and olives.

Bake the pizzas for 15 to 17 minutes until the cheese is bubbling. Serve hot.

Refrigerate leftovers in an airtight container for up to 3 days.

YIELD

12 MINI PIZZAS

NUTRITIONAL ANALYSIS

PER SERVING (1 PIZZA):

40 CALORIES

2G FAT

3G PROTEIN

3G CARBOHYDRATE

1G DIETARY FIBER

NOTE

When purchasing tomato products, look for options with no added sugar in a glass jar. The jury is still out on what chemicals are safe to use in tin cans, so choosing glass takes the guesswork out of it.

ADD IT!

These pizza bites are equally good made with pesto rather than tomato sauce. Make my Pecan Arugula Pesto (page 145) to use, or find a store-bought vegan option made with clean ingredients.

PEGAN TRAIL MIX

Make your own healthy trail mix to have on hand when hunger strikes. I like to use freeze-dried fruit in trail mix because it has a fun crunch and typically doesn't have added sugar, whereas dried fruit often does. Pack this in single-serving containers so it's just as convenient as grabbing a protein bar when you're on the run.

½ cup (73 g) almonds

½ cup (68 g) hazelnuts

½ cup (56 g) pecans

¼ cup (32 g) pumpkin seeds

3½ ounces (100 g) 70% to 90% dark chocolate, chopped

1 ounce (28 g) freeze-dried blueberries

1 ounce (28 g) freeze-dried raspberries

In a medium bowl, stir together all the trail mix ingredients, mixing well. For maximum convenience, portion into single-serving bags or containers. Store in an airtight container at room temperature for 2 to 3 months, or freezer for up to 1 year.

YIELD

8 SERVINGS

NUTRITIONAL ANALYSIS

PER SERVING (¼ CUP, OR 31 G):

156 CALORIES

12G FAT

3G PROTEIN

11G CARBOHYDRATE

3G DIETARY FIBER

NOTE

Although fresh produce is always best when it comes to nutrient density, freeze-dried fruit maintains up to 90 percent of its nutritional content, making it a great option when you need a quick or portable snack. The blueberries and raspberries in this mix add a great sweet-tart flavor.

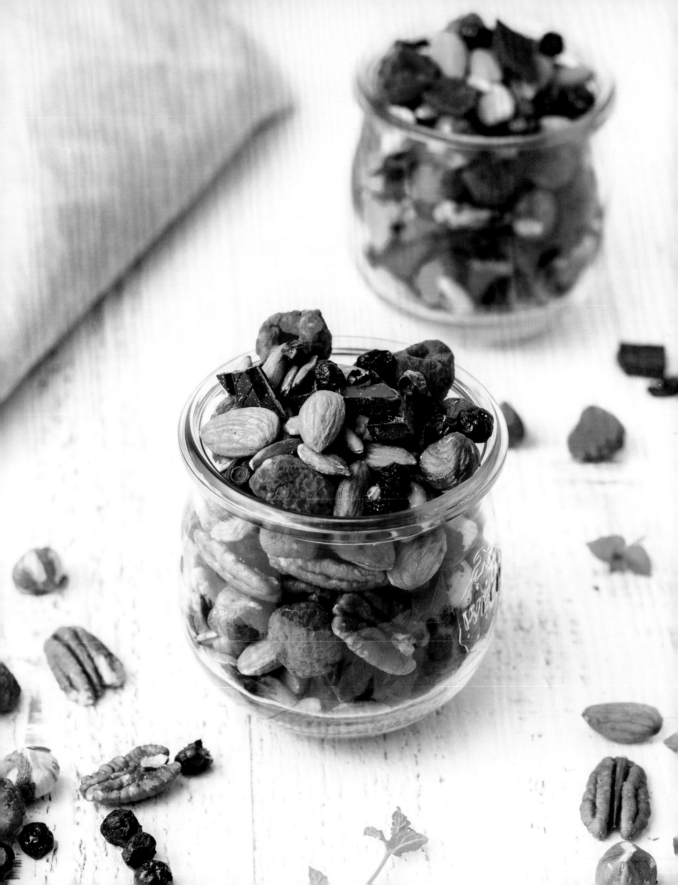

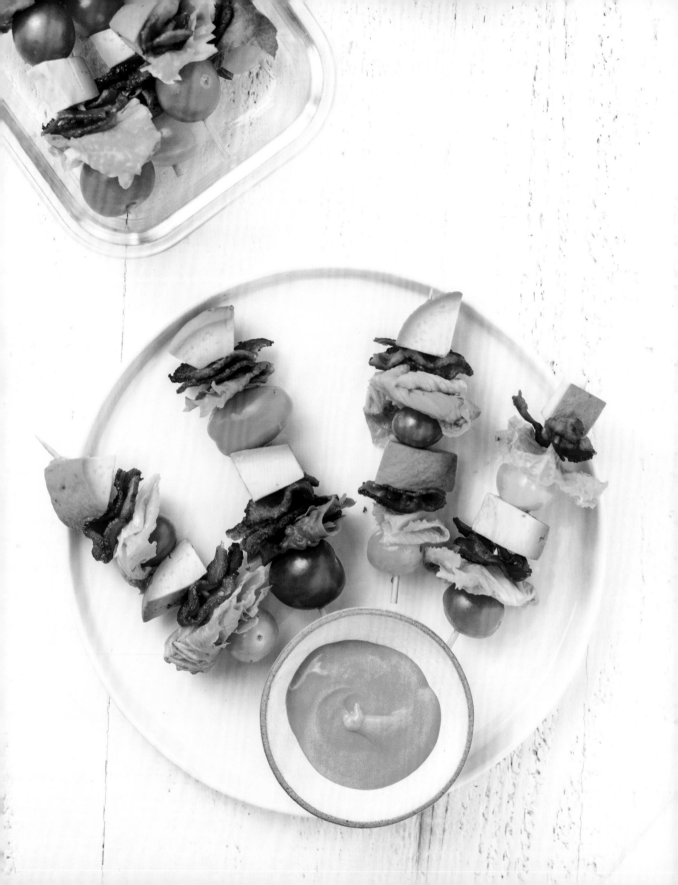

BLTA SKEWERS

Here is everyone's favorite sandwich in fun skewer form. The inside of the sandwich is the best part anyway, so ditch the bread and skewer up the veggies and bacon. These are easy to prep and keep on hand and taste just as delicious a day or two after they are made. I like to serve these with Dijon mustard or Coconut Ranch Dressing (page 153) for dipping.

8 nitrate- and nitrite-free bacon slices

4 romaine lettuce leaves, quartered (16 pieces total)

16 cherry tomatoes

1 large avocado, peeled, halved, pitted, and cut into 16 chunks

Cook the bacon to your preferred doneness. The bacon will skewer more easily if it's not too crisp. Place the bacon on paper towels to drain the grease and then cut each slice in half.

Using 8 mini skewers, skewer ½ bacon slice, 1 piece of torn lettuce, 1 cherry tomato, and 1 chunk of avocado. Repeat. Serve immediately with a dip, as desired, or refrigerate in an airtight container for up to 3 days for grab-and-go snacks.

ADD IT!

Make these even faster by subbing leftover cooked steak, chicken, or pork for the bacon. Add some extra tang by skewering pickled peppers along with the veggies. Use this basic idea, but add veggies you have on hand that need to be used. You might be surprised at how many veggies your family consumes when skewered along with pieces of bacon and served with a dip.

YIELD

8 SKEWERS

NUTRITIONAL ANALYSIS

PER SERVING (1 SKEWER):

140 CALORIES

12G FAT

4G PROTEIN

4G CARBOHYDRATE

2G DIETARY FIBER

BARBECUE KALE CHIPS

Kale is a popular veggie at the moment, and for good reason. It's one of the most nutrient-dense foods on the planet. Add some simple seasonings and bake the leaves until crunchy and an addictive snack is formed. Barbecue chips were my favorite as a kid, but if your family is picky about seasonings, these are also delicious simply seasoned with sea salt.

2 tablespoons (30 ml) avocado oil, plus more for preparing the baking sheets (optional)

1 bunch (about 7 ounces, or 200 g) kale

1½ tablespoons (14 g) coconut sugar

1 teaspoon chili powder

1 teaspoon smoked paprika

½ teaspoon garlic powder

½ teaspoon onion powder

¼ teaspoon sea salt

Preheat the oven to 300°F (150°C, or gas mark 2). Prepare 2 large baking sheets by spraying them with oil or lining them with parchment paper or silicone baking mats.

Thoroughly wash the kale, then rip the leaves off the stems and into chip-size pieces. Pat the leaves dry with a towel before placing half the kale into a large bowl.

Drizzle the kale in the bowl with 1 tablespoon (15 ml) of the oil and use your hands to massage and coat the kale with the oil.

In a small bowl, stir together the coconut sugar, chili powder, paprika, garlic power, onion powder, and salt. Sprinkle half the seasoning mixture onto the kale in the bowl, mixing it to season the kale evenly. Evenly divide the kale chips between the prepared baking sheets, spaced in an even layer. Do not overcrowd the baking sheets or the kale won't crisp.

Bake the kale chips for 10 minutes, rotate the baking trays, and bake for 8 to 12 minutes more until they begin to look translucent—but don't let them brown. They will be crispy, not soggy. Check the kale after 8 minutes to see if it's dried out enough or needs more time—once it's done, it will burn quickly. Repeat with the remaining kale, oil, and seasoning mixture.

YIELD

8 SERVINGS

NUTRITIONAL ANALYSIS

PER SERVING (1 CUP, OR 30 G):

49 CALORIES

4G FAT

1G PROTEIN

4G CARBOHYDRATE

1G DIETARY FIBER

NOTE

Kale chips are easy to make and bake—a lot faster than other types of vegetable chips. Prepare trays of kale chips to keep on the kitchen counter to make snacking healthier. If you're not sure your family will enjoy this snack, try it. A lot of kids love snacking on these salty-sweet chips.

CHAPTER 4

SOUPS AND SALADS

Eating soups and salads is a great way to increase your veggie intake. These recipes are perfect for serving as a starter to a larger meal, but also make wonderful light meals on their own. I like to make soups and salads a part of my weekly meal prep, so I have enticing veggie-rich options ready to go when my family is hungry.

CHEESY BROCCOLI CAULIFLOWER SOUP

This soup is a true indulgence. The classic recipe relies on heavy cream for its rich base, but this lightened version uses puréed cauliflower for an equally delicious but more nutritious option. Feel free to leave the broccoli chunky, as is my preference, or blend it smooth if that's more appealing to you.

1 tablespoon (15 ml) avocado oil

1 large yellow onion, chopped

2 garlic cloves, minced

4 cups (400 g) chopped cauliflower

2½ cups (600 ml) Waste-Not Vegetable Broth (page 139) or store-bought broth

8 ounces (237 g) raw Cheddar cheese, shredded

4 cups (284 g) finely chopped broccoli

1 teaspoon Dijon mustard

Pinch cayenne pepper

Sea salt and black pepper to taste

Heat a large soup pot over medium heat. Pour in the oil and add the onion and garlic. Sauté for 5 to 7 minutes to soften the vegetables. Add the cauliflower and vegetable broth, cover the pot, and cook for about 15 minutes until the cauliflower is very soft. Transfer to a blender and process until a very smooth cauliflower cream forms.

Add the Cheddar cheese and process until combined. Return the soup to the pot.

Stir in the broccoli and Dijon. Bring the soup to a low simmer, then season with cayenne and salt and black pepper to taste. Cook for about 5 minutes until the broccoli is tender. Serve hot.

Refrigerate leftover soup in an airtight container for up to 4 days,

YIELD

4 SERVINGS

NUTRITIONAL ANALYSIS

PER SERVING (1½ CUPS, OR 360 ML):

337 CALORIES

23G FAT

19G PROTEIN

17G CARBOHYDRATE

5G DIETARY FIBER

NOTE

Although most dairy products aren't recommended on the pegan diet, some raw cheeses are okay in moderation. Raw cheeses introduce good bacteria into the gut and contain digestive enzymes, meaning even some people who are lactose intolerant can enjoy them.

ADD IT!

Serve up some extra veggie goodness by adding 1 cup (120 g) finely chopped carrot, 1 cup (150 g) chopped red bell pepper, or 1 cup (70 g) thinly sliced mushrooms with the broccoli.

GREEN GAZPACHO

Gazpacho is a chilled Spanish soup made with lots of olive oil and plenty of fresh vegetables. This green version has a mild heat and silky texture—and is dairy-free, using cashew butter. It's the perfect summertime soup; there's no need to cook anything—it's made in minutes using a blender and it bursts with the season's best produce.

FOR CASHEW CREMA:

⅓ cup (86 g) raw cashew butter

⅓ cup (80 ml) water

1 tablespoon (15 ml) fresh lemon juice

1 tablespoon (15 ml) white wine vinegar

¼ teaspoon sea salt

FOR GREEN GAZPACHO:

¼ cup (60 ml) white wine vinegar

¼ cup (65 g) raw cashew butter

¼ cup (60 ml) olive oil

3 tablespoons (45 ml) fresh lime juice, plus more for seasoning

1 English cucumber, seeded and chopped

1 green bell pepper, seeded and chopped

1 pound (454 g) green heirloom tomatoes, quartered

2 lacinato kale leaves, roughly chopped

1 or 2 jalapeño peppers, seeded and chopped

2 garlic cloves, grated, plus more for seasoning

¾ teaspoon sea salt, plus more for seasoning

6 tablespoons (48 g) pistachios (optional)

1 tablespoon (8 g) sesame seeds (optional)

Paprika, for garnish (optional)

To make the cashew crema: In a blender, combine all the crema ingredients and process until a light, smooth cream forms. Transfer to a bowl and set aside to garnish the soup. Clean the blender to make the soup.

To make the green gazpacho: In a blender, combine the vinegar, cashew butter, oil, and lime juice. Process to form a creamy base.

Add the cucumber, green bell pepper, tomatoes, kale, and jalapeño(s). Process for 1 to 2 minutes until a very smooth soup forms.

Season the soup with the grated garlic and salt and process to combine. Taste and add more salt, lime juice, or garlic, as desired.

Chill the soup for at least 1 hour before serving. The flavors in this soup intensify and get even better the next day, so make it a day in advance, if you have time.

Serve the cold soup, garnished with the cashew crema, pistachios (if using), sesame seeds (if using), and a sprinkle of paprika (if using).

YIELD

6 SERVINGS

NUTRITIONAL ANALYSIS

PER SERVING (1 CUP, OR 240 ML) SOUP PLUS 2 TABLESPOONS, OR 30 G, CASHEW CREMA (DOES NOT INCLUDE OPTIONAL GARNISHES):

271 CALORIES

22G FAT

7G PROTEIN

17G CARBOHYDRATE

2G DIETARY FIBER

NOTE

Traditionally, gazpacho is made by soaking bread in an oil and vinegar mixture and blending it with lots of tomatoes and bell peppers. This version uses the creamy cashew base to keep the soup satiating, but with nutrient-dense ingredients.

CREAMY TOMATO-BASIL SOUP

This plant-powered tomato soup gets its creaminess from a rich cashew-cauliflower cream sauce. Many store-bought soups rely on starch to add thickness and sugar to add sweetness, but this soup relies on whole food ingredients instead. I like to make a double batch of this soup and freeze individual portions for quick lunches. Serve with Garlic and Rosemary Almond Meal Flaxseed Crackers (page 40) for a complete meal.

½ cup (70 g) raw cashews

3 cups (300 g) chopped cauliflower

1 tablespoon (15 ml) avocado oil

½ cup (80 g) chopped onion

3 garlic cloves, minced

1 carrot, chopped

1 (32-ounce, or 908 g) jar diced tomatoes, undrained

2¼ to 3 cups (540 to 720 ml) water, divided

1 tablespoon (6 g) vegetable bouillon

½ cup (20 g) chopped fresh basil

¼ teaspoon red pepper flakes, plus more for seasoning

Sea salt and black pepper to taste

Soak the cashews in water and cover overnight. When ready to use, drain and rinse the cashews. If there isn't enough time to soak them overnight, soak them in boiling water for 1 hour.

Place a steamer basket in a large pot and add 1 inch (2.5 cm) of water to the pot. Place the pot over medium-high heat. Place the cauliflower in the basket, cover, and steam for about 15 minutes until very soft. Drain.

In a large soup pot over medium heat, heat the oil. Add the onion, garlic, and carrot. Sauté for about 10 minutes until the vegetables are softened. Stir in the tomatoes and their juices, 1½ cups (360 ml) of the water, and the vegetable bouillon. Simmer for 5 to 10 minutes.

In a blender, combine the steamed cauliflower, drained cashews, and ¾ cup (180 ml) of water. Process for 2 to 3 minutes, or until very smooth and creamy. Remove and reserve ⅓ cup (80 ml) of cashew cream for swirling, if desired.

Add the tomato mixture to the cashew cream in the blender. Process until smooth and creamy. Add the basil and red pepper flakes and pulse until the basil is broken up. Return the soup to the pot and rewarm.

Taste and season with salt, black pepper, and red pepper flakes to taste. Thin with the remaining ¾ cup (180 ml) water if necessary. Serve the soup with a swirl of the reserved cashew cream, if desired.

YIELD

4 SERVINGS

NUTRITIONAL ANALYSIS

PER SERVING (2 CUPS, OR 480 ML):

193 CALORIES

11G FAT

7G PROTEIN

21G CARBOHYDRATE

5G DIETARY FIBER

NOTE

Buy organic tomatoes in a glass jar to avoid toxins found in cans. Whole tomatoes, crushed tomatoes, or diced tomatoes all work in this recipe.

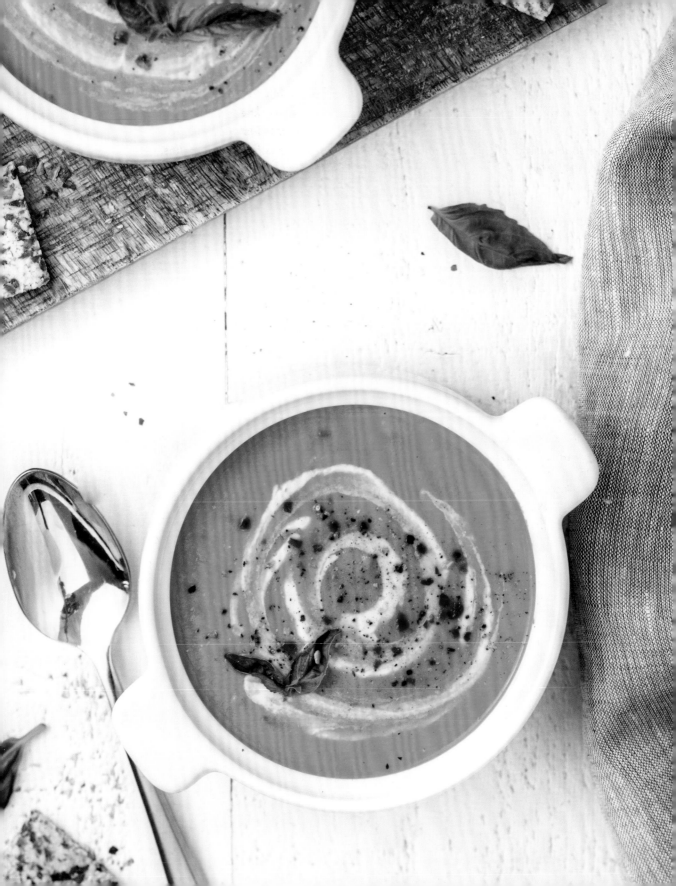

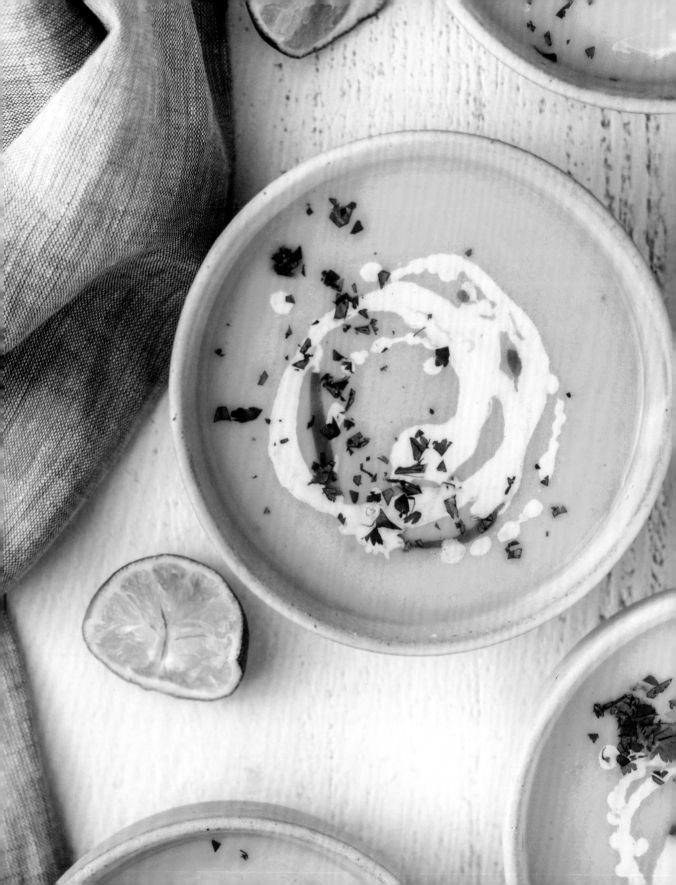

THAI-INSPIRED BUTTERNUT SOUP

Bring your favorite take-out flavors into the kitchen with this easy, soul-satisfying soup. This version uses simple, fresh ingredients, so the flavors of Thailand shine through. Creamy, sweet, and spicy, with a fresh pop of citrus, this soup will become a new favorite. I love to freeze the leftovers to reheat for quick meals.

2 (4-inch, or 10 cm) pieces lemongrass

1 (about 3-pound, or 1.4 kg) butternut squash

1 tablespoon (15 ml) sesame oil

1 large shallot, minced

⅓ cup (33 g) sliced peeled fresh ginger

3 cups (720 ml) Waste-Not Vegetable Broth (page 139) or store-bought broth

1 cup (240 ml) coconut milk

Juice of 2 large limes

½ teaspoon sea salt

1 to 3 teaspoons (5 to 15 ml) paleo sriracha

Chopped fresh cilantro, for garnish

Prepare the lemongrass by peeling off the outer "woody" layer, then thinly chopping the stalks.

Peel the butternut squash, halve it, then remove the seeds. Chop the squash into 1-inch (2.5 cm) cubes. Set aside.

In a large soup pot over medium heat, combine the oil, lemongrass, shallot, and ginger. Sauté for 5 to 7 minutes until softened and fragrant.

Add the butternut squash and vegetable broth. Simmer the soup for 15 minutes, or until the squash is very soft. Carefully transfer the soup to a blender, working in batches if needed, and process until a very creamy purée forms. Return the soup to the pot.

Stir in the coconut milk and lime juice. Bring the soup back to a low simmer, taste, and season with the salt and sriracha, as needed. Serve garnished with fresh cilantro.

YIELD

6 SERVINGS

NUTRITIONAL ANALYSIS

PER SERVING (1½ CUPS, OR 360 ML):

198 CALORIES

11G FAT

3G PROTEIN

28G CARBOHYDRATE

4G DIETARY FIBER

NOTE

If you can't find fresh lemongrass, it's often available as a paste in a jar. Asian import stores and health food stores carry lemongrass with the fresh herbs. Fresh lemongrass will have the most vibrant flavor and will be the cleanest option.

ADD IT!

Experiment by making this soup with different winter squashes. Kabocha or sugar pumpkins are great options when seasonally available.

DAIRY-FREE CORN CHOWDER

Sweet corn on the cob is one of the simple pleasures of summertime. Enjoy it on a chilly summer evening in this delicious creamy soup. Omit the bacon if you're looking for a meatless meal, but it adds a delicious smoky flavor.

½ cup (70 g) cashews

2 pounds (908 g) cauliflower florets

8 nitrate- and nitrite-free bacon slices

3 cups (720 ml) Waste-Not Vegetable Broth (page 139) or store-bought broth, divided

1 yellow onion, minced

1 cup (100 g) chopped celery

1 green bell pepper, seeded and chopped

2 carrots, chopped

2 ears sweet corn, husked and kernels cut from the cob

1 tablespoon (3 g) dried thyme, or ¼ cup (10 g) fresh thyme leaves

½ teaspoon red pepper flakes

Sea salt and black pepper to taste

Chopped scallions, for garnish (optional)

Soak the cashews in water and cover overnight. When ready to start the soup, drain and rinse the cashews and discard the water.

Place a steamer basket in a large pot and add 1 inch (2.5 cm) of water to the pot. Place the pot over medium-high heat. Place the cauliflower in the basket, cover, and steam for 15 minutes, or until very soft. The cauliflower needs to be very soft to create the silky base for the soup. Drain.

In a skillet over medium heat, fry the bacon until crisp. Reserve 2 to 3 tablespoons (30 to 45 ml) of bacon fat and 3 bacon slices to use as a garnish for the soup.

Transfer the steamed cauliflower and drained cashews to a blender, along with 1 cup (240 ml) of the vegetable broth. Process for 2 to 3 minutes until a silky, creamy sauce forms. Set aside.

Drain the steaming water from the soup pot and add the reserved bacon grease. Place the pot over medium heat and add the onion and celery. Sauté for about 5 minutes. Add the green bell pepper, carrots, and remaining 2 cups (480 ml) of vegetable broth. Simmer the mixture for about 10 minutes.

Meanwhile, chop 5 of the bacon slices.

Stir the cauliflower cream sauce into the soup pot along with the chopped bacon and sweet corn. Season with the thyme, red pepper flakes, and salt and black pepper to taste. Taste and adjust the seasonings.

Serve the soup garnished with the reserved bacon, chopped, and scallions (if using).

YIELD

6 SERVINGS

NUTRITIONAL ANALYSIS

PER SERVING (1½ CUPS, OR 360 ML):

248 CALORIES

17G FAT

9G PROTEIN

18G CARBOHYDRATE

5G DIETARY FIBER

NOTE

You can use ¼ cup (65 g) cashew butter as a quick substitute for the soaked cashews. If you forget to soak the cashews ahead, keeping a jar of cashew butter on hand is an easy solution. Add the cashew butter to the blender along with the steamed cauliflower.

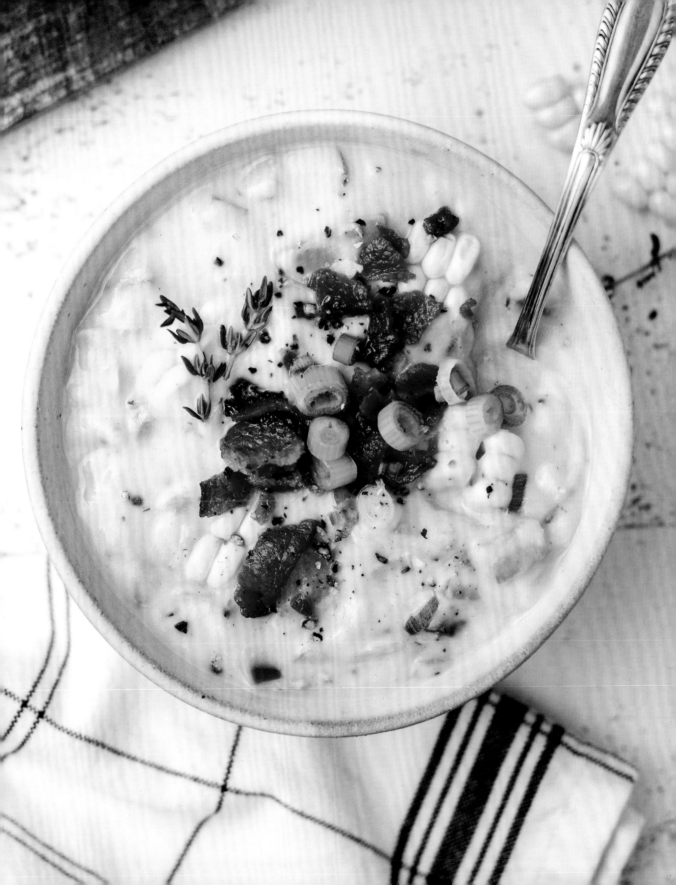

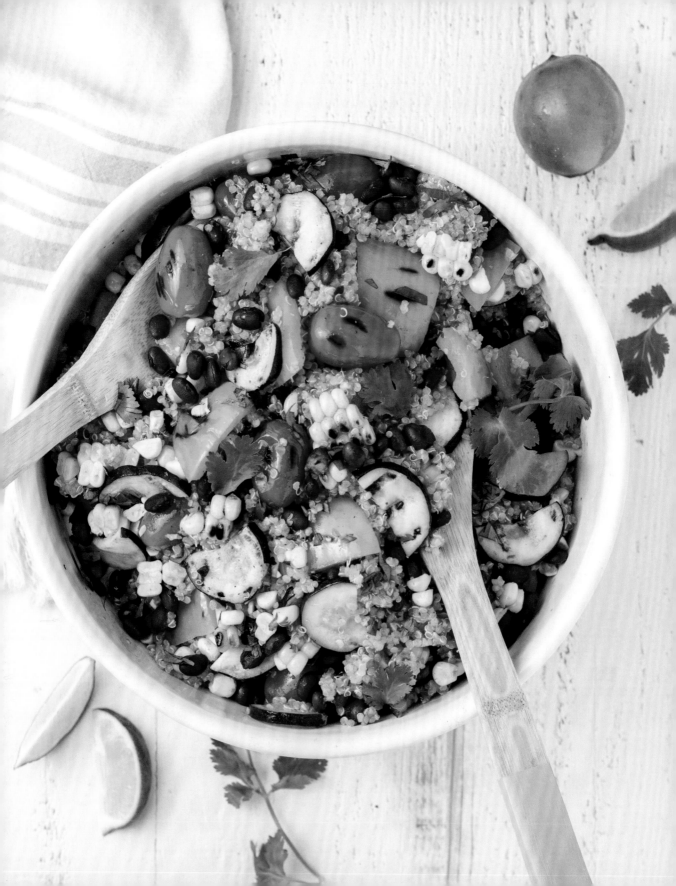

MEXICAN QUINOA SALAD WITH GRILLED VEGETABLES

This is a delicious salad that's perfect for a prep-ahead option. It's flavorful with hot vegetables right off the grill, but I typically grill the vegetables and prep the quinoa and dressing ahead, then mix everything when I am ready to serve. This salad is heavy on vegetables and a perfect summer side to a cookout.

FOR SALSA VINAIGRETTE:

¾ cup (195 g) salsa

6 tablespoons (90 ml) red wine vinegar

¼ cup (60 ml) olive oil

1 teaspoon ground cumin

½ teaspoon sea salt, or to taste

FOR QUINOA SALAD:

½ cup (92 g) raw quinoa, cooked according to package directions

1 (15-ounce, or 425 g) can black beans, rinsed and drained

2 bell peppers, any color, cut into 1-inch (2.5 cm) squares

1 zucchini, cut into thick slices

1 cup (149 g) cherry tomatoes

1 tablespoon (15 ml) olive oil, plus more for the corn

Sea salt and black pepper to taste

1 ear corn, husked and silks removed

½ cup (8 g) chopped fresh cilantro

To make the salsa vinaigrette: In a blender, combine all the vinaigrette ingredients and pulse a few times to mix well and smooth out some of the chunkiness from the salsa. Set aside.

To make the quinoa salad: In a large salad bowl, stir together the cooked quinoa and black beans.

In a medium bowl, combine the bell peppers, zucchini, and tomatoes and drizzle with the oil. Season with salt and pepper to taste.

Spray or brush the corn with oil.

Heat an outdoor grill to medium-high heat, or heat a grill pan over medium-high heat. Add the vegetables and cook for 3 to 5 minutes per side, long enough to have soft grill marks, being careful not to burn them.

Cut the corn kernels from the cob and add them to the quinoa and black beans. Add the remaining grilled vegetables and mix well to combine.

Add the cilantro and the salsa vinaigrette to the salad bowl and toss to combine and coat.

YIELD

8 SERVINGS

NUTRITIONAL ANALYSIS

PER SERVING (1 CUP, OR ABOUT 200 G):

177 CALORIES

8G FAT

6G PROTEIN

22G CARBOHYDRATE

5G DIETARY FIBER

ADD IT!

Experiment with the grilled veggies in this delicious salad. Eggplant, asparagus, and mushrooms are all great options for grilling.

SUMMER GREEK SALAD

Punch up your Greek salad with a summery twist. Greek salads are loaded with fresh, nutrient-dense vegetables, and the traditional olive oil and vinegar dressing is both the simplest and healthiest way to dress a salad. This version has a sweet pop from sliced nectarines and features a robust basil-mint dressing. Add quinoa to turn this into a complete meal, or serve alongside grilled meats for a light summery dinner.

FOR SALAD:

4 cups (80 g) arugula

2 cups (360 g) diced (1-inch, or 2.5 cm) Roma tomatoes

2 nectarines, pitted and sliced

1 cup (155 g) pitted black olives

1 English cucumber, sliced and quartered

½ cup (80 g) sliced red onion

½ cup (60 g) chopped walnuts

FOR BASIL-MINT VINAIGRETTE:

6 tablespoons (90 ml) olive oil

⅓ cup (32 g) fresh mint

⅓ cup (13 g) fresh basil

3 tablespoons (45 ml) fresh lemon juice

3 tablespoons (45 ml) red wine vinegar

1 tablespoon (20 g) maple syrup

2 teaspoons Dijon mustard

1 teaspoon minced garlic

¼ teaspoon sea salt

Black pepper to taste

To make the salad: In a large salad bowl, gently mix the arugula, tomatoes, nectarines, olives, cucumber, and red onion.

To make the vinaigrette: In a blender, combine all the dressing ingredients and process for about 30 seconds until the herbs are finely chopped.

When ready to serve, add the dressing to the salad and toss to combine and coat. Garnish with the chopped walnuts.

Refrigerate leftovers in an airtight container for up to 3 days.

YIELD

6 SERVINGS

NUTRITIONAL ANALYSIS

PER SERVING (1 CUP, OR ABOUT 200 G):

285 CALORIES

24G FAT

4G PROTEIN

17G CARBOHYDRATE

4G DIETARY FIBER

NOTE

Salads are a great way to use up fresh produce you have on hand. Substitute a different green in this salad, like baby greens or even chopped romaine lettuce. You can use peaches in place of the nectarines or chopped almonds or pecans in place of the walnuts.

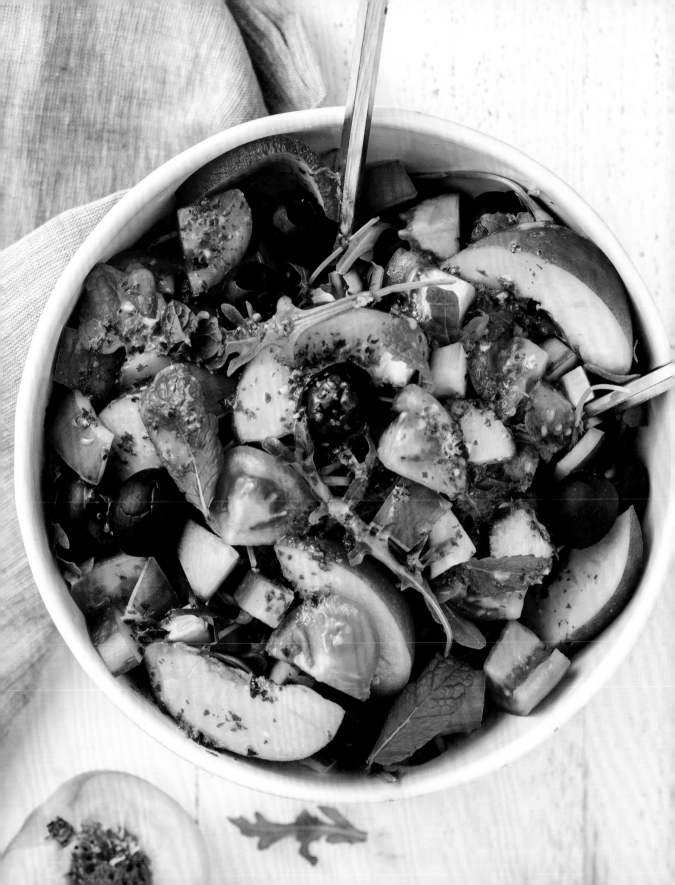

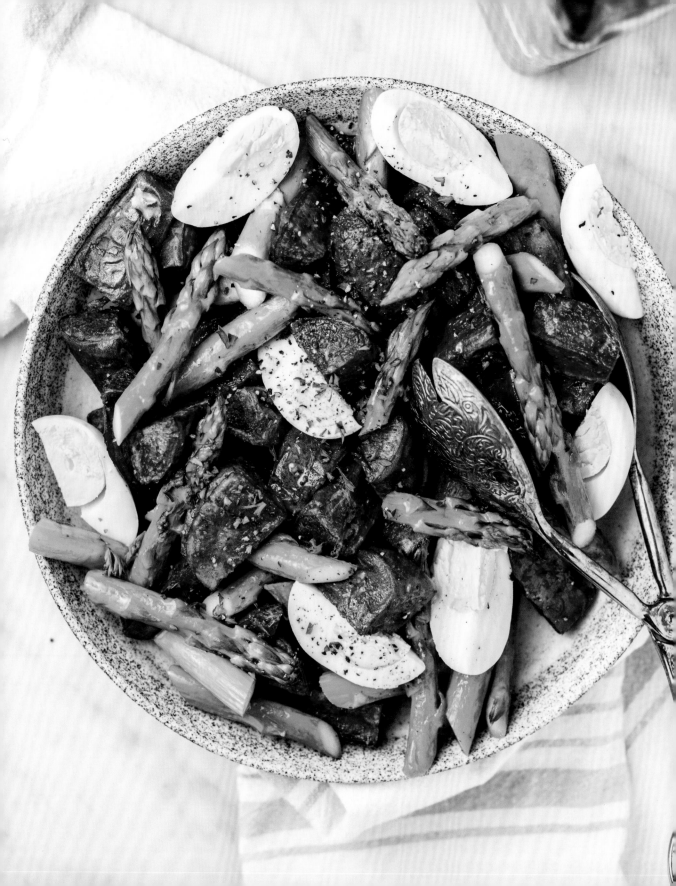

ROASTED PURPLE SWEET POTATO AND ASPARAGUS SALAD

This stunning spring salad is a refreshing twist on a classic picnic potato salad. Rather than using white potatoes, purple sweet potatoes add anthocyanins, an antioxidant found in purple-hued vegetables, as well as lots of vitamin C, potassium, and fiber. The creamy, sweet flesh is the perfect contrast to crisp asparagus and the bright lemon dressing.

3 purple sweet potatoes or white sweet potatoes, cut into 1½-inch (3.5 cm) cubes

2 tablespoons (30 ml) avocado oil, divided

Sea salt and black pepper to taste

1 pound (454 g) asparagus, woody ends trimmed, cut into 1-inch (2.5 cm) pieces

4 large eggs, hard-boiled, peeled, and quartered

Chopped fresh parsley, for garnish

½ cup (120 ml) Easy Lemon Vinaigrette (page 148)

Preheat the oven to 425°F (220°C, or gas mark 7).

On a large baking sheet, arrange the purple sweet potatoes. Drizzle with 1 tablespoon (15 ml) of the oil and season with salt and pepper to taste.

Bake for 20 minutes.

Add the asparagus to the baking sheet, drizzling it with the remaining 1 tablespoon (15 ml) of oil. Return to the oven and roast for 7 to 10 minutes more until the asparagus is crisp-tender.

Transfer the hot vegetables to a serving platter and arrange the hard-boiled eggs with the vegetables. Garnish with fresh parsley.

Drizzle the salad with the vinaigrette. Serve hot or cold.

Refrigerate leftovers in an airtight container for up to 4 days.

YIELD

8 SERVINGS

NUTRITIONAL ANALYSIS

PER SERVING (1 CUP, OR ABOUT 150 G):

162 CALORIES

11G FAT

3G PROTEIN

13G CARBOHYDRATE

3G DIETARY FIBER

NOTE

Purple sweet potatoes have a much lower glycemic index (24) than white russet potatoes (111), making them a better choice for managing blood sugar levels. Look for them near the sweet potatoes and yams, or find them at a specialty grocery store.

CROWD-PLEASING BROCCOLI SALAD

Serve up everyone's favorite veggie in this healthy salad. Rather than mayo, the broccoli is tossed in a healthy creamy tahini dressing. Tahini adds an extra dose of fiber and protein along with nutrients that reduce heart disease risk and inflammation. This salad is high enough in protein to serve as a light lunch. It is also a great side dish for family dinners. When attending picnics and potlucks, I always bring a healthy veggie-heavy dish, and this salad disappears quickly.

FOR CREAMY TAHINI DRESSING:

¼ cup (60 g) tahini

¼ cup (60 ml) olive oil

¼ cup (60 ml) fresh lemon juice

¼ cup (60 ml) white wine vinegar

1 tablespoon (20 g) maple syrup

2 teaspoons Dijon mustard

¼ teaspoon sea salt

Black pepper to taste

FOR BROCCOLI SALAD:

8 cups (568 g) chopped broccoli

1 pound (454 g) bacon, cooked until crisp, drained

1 yellow bell pepper, seeded and chopped

½ cup (80 g) finely chopped red onion

½ cup (70 g) roasted cashews

To make the creamy tahini dressing: In a jar or blender, combine all the dressing ingredients. Cover the jar and shake or process to combine into a creamy dressing. I prefer to use a blender because it adds air to the dressing and makes it light and ultra-creamy.

To make the broccoli salad: Place the broccoli in a large bowl and drizzle it with the tahini dressing. Toss to coat. Refrigerate the broccoli, letting the dressing soak in, while preparing the toppings.

When ready to serve, top the salad with the bacon, yellow bell pepper, red onion, and cashews. Toss the salad to combine and coat.

For the best texture, refrigerate leftovers in an airtight container without the bacon and cashews, which will get soggy when stored overnight. If I know my family will not finish the whole salad at one meal, I toss the salad with the bell pepper and onion and pack half away. Refrigerate half the cooked bacon and store half the cashews separately to top the remaining salad the next day.

YIELD

9 SERVINGS

NUTRITIONAL ANALYSIS

PER SERVING (1 CUP, OR ABOUT 125 G):

386 CALORIES

16G FAT

11G PROTEIN

13G CARBOHYDRATE

3G DIETARY FIBER

ADD IT!

A traditional broccoli salad has raisins and red grapes. Those are both good additions but, because they have a high sugar content, should be reserved for special occasions. Raw Cheddar cheese cubes are also a delicious addition.

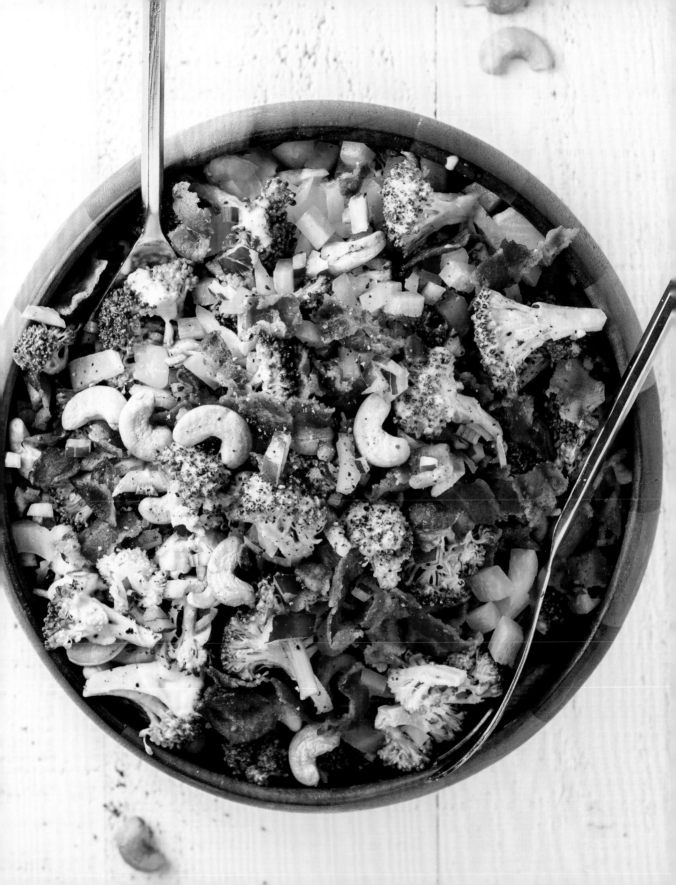

HEIRLOOM TOMATO AND HERB SALAD

Choosing produce that isn't mass-produced, like heirloom tomatoes, means it's less likely it's been genetically modified. These showstopping tomatoes make a beautiful side dish on their own. This simple salad gets its crunch from cucumber and onion and is dressed with a simple herb vinaigrette. Serve this salad all summer with whatever herbs you have growing in the garden.

FOR SALAD:

4 large (about 1½ pounds, or 568 g) heirloom tomatoes, sliced

1 English cucumber, thinly sliced

¼ cup (40 g) thinly sliced red onion

FOR HERB VINAIGRETTE:

¼ cup (60 ml) olive oil

¼ cup (60 ml) fresh lime juice

2 tablespoons (12 g) chopped fresh mint

2 tablespoons (8 g) chopped fresh dill

2 tablespoons (6 g) chopped fresh chives

¼ teaspoon sea salt

Black pepper to taste

To make the salad: On a platter, arrange the tomatoes, cucumber, and red onion, alternating to mix the vegetables.

To make the herb vinaigrette: In a small bowl, whisk all the dressing ingredients to combine. Drizzle the vinaigrette over the vegetables. Serve immediately.

Refrigerate leftovers in an airtight container for 1 to 2 days.

YIELD

8 SERVINGS

NUTRITIONAL ANALYSIS

PER SERVING (1 CUP, OR ABOUT 100 G):

99 CALORIES

7G FAT

2G PROTEIN

9G CARBOHYDRATE

2G DIETARY FIBER

NOTE

Heirloom tomatoes can be found at some specialty food stores year-round and are abundant at summer farmers' markets. They come in all shapes and sizes, so choose a colorful variety of large tomatoes or substitute 5 to 6 cups (745 to 894 g) heirloom cherry tomatoes. Even green heirloom tomatoes are ripe and taste sweet.

ADD IT!

Choose herbs growing in your garden or that you keep on hand for other recipes. Fresh cilantro, parsley, and basil are great options in this dressing.

◆ ◆ ◆

CHAPTER 5

ENTRÉES

Plan for success by choosing entrées for the week, preparing a shopping list, and prepping some of the sauces, dressings, or marinades you need.

This section has a range of simple mains, like the Speedy Chickpea and Veggie Curry (page 82), Salmon and Artichoke Skewers (page 84), and Roasted Turkey Legs with Vegetables (page 100), and some more complex meals, perfect for weekend meal prep, holidays, or special family meals.

As a part of your meal prep, you might want to choose freezable options, like the Golden Lentil Soup with Spinach and Tomatoes (page 78), the Turkey Sweet Potato Chili (page 91), or Creamy Sausage, Celeriac, and Kale Soup (page 98), so at the end of the week, you have healthy options ready to reheat.

If you choose a meat-focused entrée, add a side dish to keep your plate 75/25 (see page 17).

VEGETARIAN

MOROCCAN-STYLE
CHICKPEA SALAD | 75

WINTER GLOW
WILD RICE SALAD | 77

GOLDEN LENTIL SOUP WITH
SPINACH AND TOMATOES | 78

EGGPLANT MEATBALLS WITH
ZOODLES | 81

SPEEDY CHICKPEA
AND VEGGIE CURRY | 82

SEAFOOD

SALMON IN WATERCRESS
SAUCE | 83

SALMON AND ARTICHOKE
SKEWERS | 84

SEARED SCALLOPS IN
BROWN BUTTER SAUCE | 87

COCONUT SHRIMP | 88

DON'T FEAR CIOPPINO | 90

POULTRY

TURKEY SWEET POTATO CHILI | 91

CLEANED-UP COBB SALAD | 93

TOM KHA GAI | 94

IMMUNE-BOOSTING
CHICKEN ZOODLE SOUP | 97

CREAMY SAUSAGE, CELERIAC,
AND KALE SOUP | 98

SESAME-GINGER GRILLED
CHICKEN | 99

ROASTED TURKEY LEGS
WITH VEGETABLES | 100

PORK, BEEF, AND LAMB

MAPLE-DIJON PORK TENDERLOIN
WITH WATERCRESS AND
APPLE SALAD | 102

MOJO PORK ROAST | 105

VIETNAMESE-STYLE
PORK BÁNH MÌ BOWLS | 106

GRILLED ROSEMARY PORK
SKEWERS | 108

KALE TACO SALAD | 111

SHEPHERD'S PIE WITH
CAULIFLOWER PARSNIP CRUST | 112

SEARED LAMB CHOPS
WITH CITRUS MINT SALAD | 114

BEEF RENDANG | 116

GRASS-FED ROAST BEEF | 118

MOROCCAN-STYLE CHICKPEA SALAD

This salad is a flavorful combo of roasted and fresh veggies, punctuated by Moroccan-spiced baked chickpeas. Served over a bed of quinoa and topped with lively herbs, it's bursting with fiber and nutrients.

FOR SPICED CHICKPEAS:

1 (15-ounce, or 425 g) can chickpeas, rinsed and drained

2 tablespoons (30 ml) fresh lemon juice

2 tablespoon (30 ml) avocado oil, divided

2 teaspoons ground cumin

1 teaspoon ground cinnamon

1 teaspoon paprika

¾ teaspoon sea salt

½ teaspoon ground ginger

½ teaspoon ground turmeric

⅛ teaspoon cayenne pepper

FOR ROASTED VEGETABLES:

4 cups (560 g) cubed butternut squash

2 beets, peeled and cubed

1 tablespoon (15 ml) avocado oil

Sea salt and black pepper to taste

FOR MOROCCAN SALAD:

½ cup (92 g) raw quinoa, rinsed

2 cups (298 g) halved cherry tomatoes

1 English cucumber, sliced

½ cup (8 g) chopped fresh cilantro

½ cup (30 g) chopped fresh Italian parsley

½ cup (120 ml) Easy Lemon Vinaigrette (page 148)

To make the spiced chickpeas: Preheat the oven to 425°F (220°C, or gas mark 7).

In a small bowl, stir together the chickpeas, lemon juice, 1 tablespoon (15 ml) of the oil, and seasonings until evenly coated. Spread the seasoned chickpeas in an even layer across one-third of a large sheet pan.

To make the roasted vegetables: Place the butternut squash and the beet cubes on the other two-thirds of the sheet pan. Drizzle the vegetables with the remaining oil and generously season with salt and pepper to taste.

Roast the vegetables and chickpeas for 30 minutes until the vegetables are soft and the chickpeas are crisp.

To make the salad: While the vegetables roast, cook the quinoa according to the package directions. Let cool slightly and transfer to a large salad bowl.

Add the roasted vegetables and chickpeas, tomatoes, cucumber, cilantro, and parsley. Drizzle with the lemon vinaigrette and toss to coat and combine.

YIELD

4 SERVINGS

NUTRITIONAL ANALYSIS

PER SERVING (2½ CUPS, WEIGHT VARIES):

403 CALORIES

26G FAT

7G PROTEIN

41G CARBOHYDRATE

7G DIETARY FIBER

ADD IT!

If you need a higher-protein meal but love the sound of this recipe, swap the chickpeas for 1 pound (454 g) chicken breast cut into 1-inch (2.5 cm) pieces. The chicken can be tossed in the same seasoning mix and roasted along with the vegetables. This option is better for people who have insulin sensitivity or who are trying to lose weight.

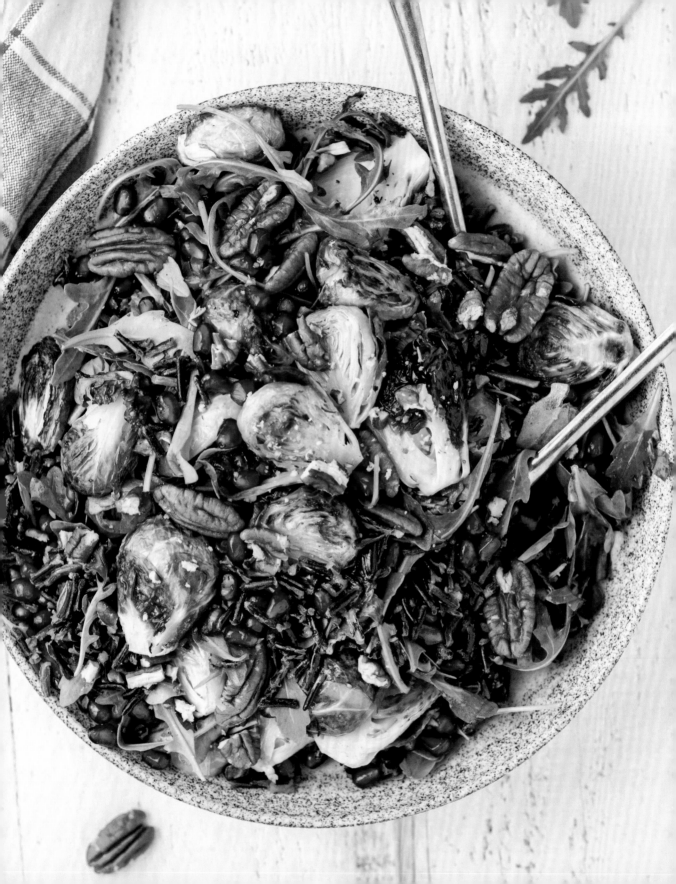

WINTER GLOW WILD RICE SALAD

Crispy roasted Brussels sprouts are the star in this fall-themed wild rice salad. This salad has a ton of tastes and textures and is sure to provide a green boost and bright flavors to a cool winter day. Omit the wild rice to make this salad even lower on the glycemic index.

FOR ROASTED BRUSSELS SPROUTS:

1 pound (454 g) Brussels sprouts, halved

1 tablespoon (15 ml) avocado oil

Sea salt and black pepper to taste

FOR WILD RICE:

½ cup (80 g) wild rice

1 cup (240 ml) Waste-Not Vegetable Broth (page 139) or store-bought broth

1 tablespoon (14 g) pastured butter

FOR WINTER GLOW SALAD:

4 cups (80 g) arugula

½ cup (120 ml) Easy Lemon Vinaigrette (page 148)

1 cup (180 g) pomegranate arils

⅓ cup (34 g) pecans, toasted

To make the roasted Brussels sprouts: Preheat the oven to 450°F (230°C, or gas mark 8).

Arrange the Brussels sprout halves on a sheet pan and drizzle with the oil. Generously season with salt and pepper and toss to coat evenly.

Bake the Brussels sprouts for 20 to 25 minutes until the outer leaves have crisped up.

To make the wild rice: In a small saucepan with a lid over high heat, combine the wild rice, vegetable broth, and butter. Bring to a boil, reduce the heat to low, and cover the pan. Cook for 30 to 40 minutes until no broth remains. Set aside to cool.

To make the salad: Once the rice has begun to cool, transfer it to a large salad bowl. Add the Brussels sprouts and arugula. Drizzle the salad with the vinaigrette and toss to coat and combine.

Garnish the salad with the pomegranate arils and toasted pecans to serve.

YIELD

4 SERVINGS

NUTRITIONAL ANALYSIS

PER SERVING (2 CUPS, OR ABOUT 200 G):

413 CALORIES

27G FAT

9G PROTEIN

40G CARBOHYDRATE

9G DIETARY FIBER

NOTE

Wild rice is not actually rice, but rather an aquatic grass. It has a chewy texture and earthy flavor, perfect for tossing in salads with tangy dressings or adding to creamy soups.

ADD IT!

Choose an in-season fruit to top this salad. Pears, apples, and orange slices are all great options.

GOLDEN LENTIL SOUP WITH SPINACH AND TOMATOES

This light yet filling vegan soup comes together in about 10 minutes, then simmers for 30 minutes. It packs a serious nutritional punch from the combination of anti-inflammatory spices, fiber-rich lentils, and satiating healthy fats in the coconut milk. As beautiful as it is delicious, this soup is perfect for meal prep. Make a batch and freeze it in individual portions or just keep it on hand in the fridge for a week to heat as needed.

1 tablespoon (15 ml) avocado oil

1 cup (160 g) minced onion

3 garlic cloves, minced

1 tablespoon (7 g) ground turmeric

1 tablespoon (7 g) ground cumin

½ teaspoon ground cinnamon

½ teaspoon ground ginger

½ teaspoon sea salt

4 cups (960 ml) Waste-Not Vegetable Broth (page 139) or store-bought broth

¾ cup (148 g) red lentils

2 cups (520 g) canned diced tomatoes (from a glass jar, if possible)

2 cups (480 ml) full-fat coconut milk

6 cups (180 g) fresh spinach

2 tablespoons (30 ml) fresh lime juice

Pinch cayenne pepper, or to taste

In a large Dutch oven or soup pot over medium heat, heat the oil. Add the onion and garlic and sauté for about 5 minutes until softened.

Add the spices and a few tablespoons (about 45 ml) of vegetable broth, as necessary, and lightly fry the spices for 2 to 3 minutes until fragrant.

Stir in the remaining vegetable broth, lentils, and tomatoes and bring the soup to a simmer. Turn the heat to medium-low and simmer the soup for 20 to 30 minutes until the lentils are soft.

Stir in the coconut milk, spinach, lime juice, and cayenne. Let the soup return to a low simmer. Once it's warmed through, remove from the heat and serve.

YIELD

6 SERVINGS

NUTRITIONAL ANALYSIS

PER SERVING (1½ CUPS, OR 360 ML):

305 CALORIES

19G FAT

10G PROTEIN

28G CARBOHYDRATE

10G DIETARY FIBER

ADD IT!

Other greens, like chopped kale, chard, or collard greens, are great additions in place of the spinach. Using 3 cups (360 g) sliced zucchini or (213 g) chopped broccoli also works beautifully in this soup.

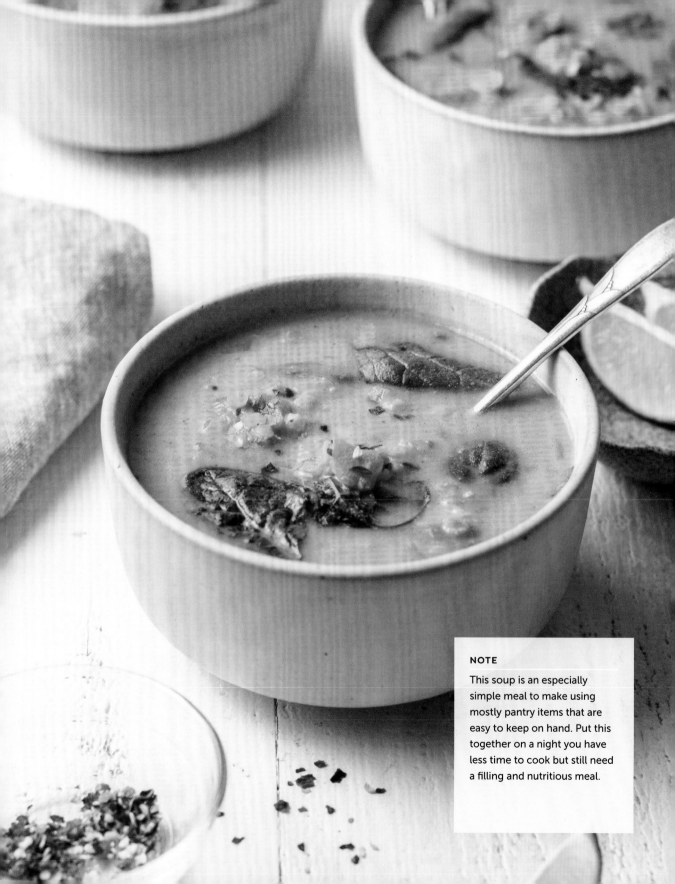

NOTE

This soup is an especially simple meal to make using mostly pantry items that are easy to keep on hand. Put this together on a night you have less time to cook but still need a filling and nutritious meal.

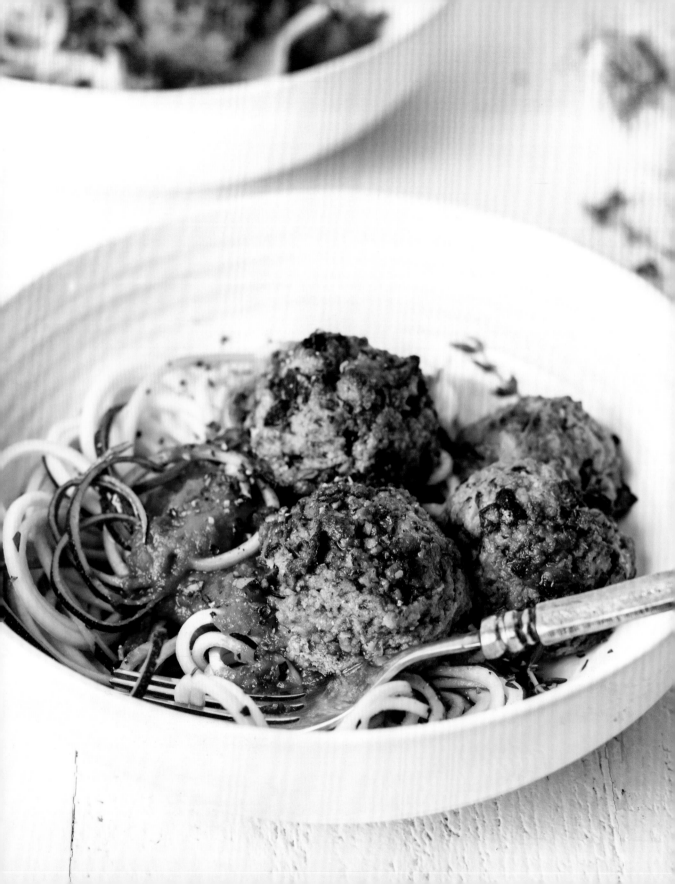

EGGPLANT MEATBALLS WITH ZOODLES

Eggplant is a delicious low-carb vegetable, high in antioxidants and fiber. Learning how to cook eggplant well is a skill. This fun eggplant "meatball" recipe is easy to make, delicious, and a great topping for a plate of zucchini noodles.

FOR EGGPLANT MEATBALLS:

1 large (about 1¼-pound, or 560 g) eggplant, cut into 1-inch (2.5 cm) cubes

1 cup (160 g) diced onion

3 garlic cloves, minced

1 tablespoon (15 ml) olive oil

Sea salt and black pepper to taste

¾ cup (72 g) almond flour

1 large egg

1 teaspoon Italian seasoning

FOR ZOODLES:

2 large zucchini

12 ounces (340 g) organic marinara sauce

YIELD

4 SERVINGS

NUTRITIONAL ANALYSIS

PER SERVING (4 EGGPLANT MEATBALLS, ½ ZUCCHINI, 3 OUNCES, OR 55 G, PASTA SAUCE):

252 CALORIES
16G FAT
10G PROTEIN
24G CARBOHYDRATE
9G DIETARY FIBER

To make the eggplant meatballs: Preheat the oven to 400°F (200°C, or gas mark 6). Line a sheet pan with parchment paper or a silicone mat. Set aside.

On a large sheet pan, combine the eggplant, onion, and garlic. Drizzle with the oil and season with salt and pepper to taste.

Bake the eggplant for 30 minutes. Reduce the oven temperature to 375°F (190°C, or gas mark 5).

Transfer the baked eggplant, onion, and garlic to a food processor and add the almond flour, egg, Italian seasoning, and ½ teaspoon of salt. Pulse 10 to 12 times until the mixture is well mixed but the eggplant is still slightly chunky. Don't form a smooth paste, but rather a chunky but sticky mixture.

Use a 2-tablespoon (30 ml) cookie or ice-cream scoop to portion the eggplant mixture onto the prepared sheet pan. Wetting the scoop with water before scooping helps the mixture come out more easily.

Bake the meatballs for 40 minutes until they begin to crisp up on the outside.

To make the zoodles: Spiralize the zucchini and divide it among the plates raw.

Heat the marinara sauce until very hot and top the zoodles with it right before serving. This will heat up the dish without overcooking the zoodles, which makes them watery.

Top the zoodles and marinara sauce with the meatballs.

NOTE

If you don't have a spiralizer for the zucchini noodles, use a vegetable peeler to make long strands of squash. Another low-cost option for making vegetable noodles is to use a julienne peeler.

SPEEDY CHICKPEA AND VEGGIE CURRY

This recipe can be made with any variety of veggies you have on hand and a few cans from your pantry. Recipes like this are essential for getting through busy weeks. My family loves this flavorful curry served over cauliflower rice or quinoa.

1 tablespoon (15 ml) avocado oil

½ cup (80 g) diced onion

4 garlic cloves, minced

4 cups (400 g) diced veggies (I use carrots, bell pepper, and zucchini)

1 (15-ounce, or 425 g) can chickpeas, rinsed and drained

1 (18-ounce, or 509 g) jar diced tomatoes

2 cups (480 ml) coconut milk

1 tablespoon (6 g) curry powder, plus more for seasoning

1 teaspoon sea salt, plus more for seasoning

In a large skillet or Dutch oven over medium heat, combine the oil, onion, and garlic. Sauté for about 10 minutes until softened.

Add the diced veggies and cook for about 5 more minutes, stirring, to soften.

Stir in the chickpeas, tomatoes, coconut milk, curry powder, and salt. Turn the heat to medium-low and simmer the curry for 10 minutes until the veggies are crisp-tender. Taste and adjust the seasonings as needed.

YIELD

4 SERVINGS

NUTRITIONAL ANALYSIS

PER SERVING (1 CUP, OR ABOUT 275 G):

316 CALORIES

28G FAT

5G PROTEIN

17G CARBOHYDRATE

4G DIETARY FIBER

NOTE

If you don't have curry powder, substitute 1 teaspoon each of paprika, ground turmeric, ground ginger and a few pinches of cayenne pepper to taste.

ADD IT!

This recipe works well with red lentils in place of the chickpeas. Add ½ cup (98 g) dried red lentils to the curry with the tomatoes and coconut milk and extend the cook time to 20 to 25 minutes to allow them to soften fully.

SALMON IN WATERCRESS SAUCE

A simple baked salmon dish is elevated by a flavorful green sauce, kept creamy and nutrient packed using my favorite nut, cashews. This dish is especially comforting on a chilly winter night when short, less-active days zap your energy. Watercress is one of the most nutrient-dense greens and can be incorporated into meals fresh or used in soups and sauces.

FOR BAKED SALMON:

4 (4-ounce, or 225 g) wild salmon fillets

1 tablespoon (15 ml) avocado oil

Sea salt and black pepper to taste

FOR WATERCRESS SAUCE:

1 tablespoon (14 g) pastured butter

2 small shallots, minced

1 cup (240 ml) fish stock

¼ cup (65 g) cashew butter

3 cups (136 g) watercress

2 tablespoons (30 ml) fresh lemon juice

¼ cup (16 g) chopped fresh dill

Sea salt and black pepper to taste

To make the salmon: Preheat the oven to 425°F (220°C).

Place the salmon fillets on a sheet pan and drizzle with the oil. Season with salt and pepper to taste.

Bake the salmon for 12 to 16 minutes, depending on the desired doneness. Twelve minutes results in a medium-rare salmon; 16 minutes will be closer to fully cooked. Serve the salmon with the watercress sauce.

To make the watercress sauce: While the salmon bakes, in a large skillet over medium heat, melt the butter. Add the shallots and sauté for about 7 minutes until translucent. Stir in the fish stock. Simmer for about 10 minutes until reduced by half.

Stir in the cashew butter and watercress. Cover the skillet and cook for no more than 2 minutes to wilt the watercress. Transfer to a blender and add the lemon juice and dill. Process to form a bright green, creamy sauce. Return the sauce to the skillet. Taste and season with salt and pepper, as needed.

YIELD

4 SERVINGS

NUTRITIONAL ANALYSIS

PER SERVING (1 SALMON FILLET AND ½ CUP, OR 120 ML, WATERCRESS SAUCE):

331 CALORIES

22G FAT

27G PROTEIN

7G CARBOHYDRATE

1G DIETARY FIBER

NOTE

The sustainability of our oceans is threatened by pollution and overfishing. Support companies that ethically harvest seafood. The Marine Stewardship Council is a watchdog for the fisheries industry. You can look for seafood that's earned the MSC label to know you're supporting companies working to protect our oceans.

ADD IT!

Serve this meal with an extra dose of veggies. I recommend pairing this with Roasted Purple Sweet Potato and Asparagus Salad (page 69) or, in summer, Heirloom Tomato and Herb Salad (page 72).

SALMON AND ARTICHOKE SKEWERS

These delicious skewers are perfect for summer cookouts, but I also bake these in the oven during cooler months. When grilling, use a lower temperature to prevent overly charring the salmon, which will reduce the amount of harmful compounds that form when cooking over high heat or a flame. These are the perfect meal on their own, but also delicious served over rice or cauliflower rice.

1 pound (454 g) salmon, cut into 1-inch (2.5 cm) cubes

1 lemon, thinly sliced into rounds

1 (14-ounce, or 400 g) can artichoke hearts in water, drained and halved

3 bell peppers (1 red, 1 yellow, 1 green), cut into 1-inch (2.5 cm) squares

½ large red onion, cut into 1-inch (2.5 cm) squares

1 tablespoon (15 ml) avocado oil

Sea salt and black pepper to taste

Chimichurri (page 144), for serving

Prepare 16 skewers by soaking them in water for at least 10 minutes, or up to 1 hour, before skewering the salmon and vegetables.

Preheat a grill to medium heat.

Using 8 skewers, skewer the salmon, alternating with folded lemon rounds.

On the remaining 8 skewers, alternate artichoke hearts, bell pepper, and red onion.

Brush the skewers with the oil and season with salt and pepper to taste.

Grill the skewers for 5 minutes per side, or until the salmon is cooked through and flakes easily with a fork. Serve with chimichurri for drizzling.

YIELD

4 SERVINGS

NUTRITIONAL ANALYSIS

PER SERVING (2 SALMON SKEWERS AND 2 VEGETABLE SKEWERS):

238 CALORIES

11G FAT

25G PROTEIN

9G CARBOHYDRATE

2G DIETARY FIBER

NOTE

If you're particularly worried about the formation of compounds caused when grilling meats, wrap the skewers in aluminum foil. I often do this and make these "deconstructed," placing the bell pepper, onion, artichokes, and salmon in a foil pouch rather than on skewers.

ADD IT!

A variety of veggies work well on these skewers, such as zucchini, olives, cherry tomatoes, asparagus, and even fruit like peaches or pineapple.

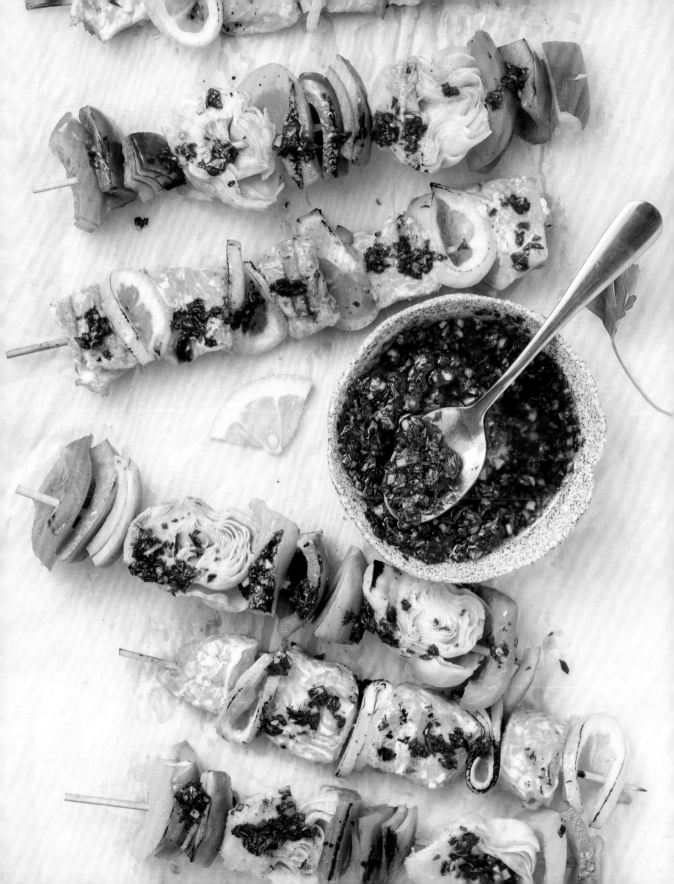

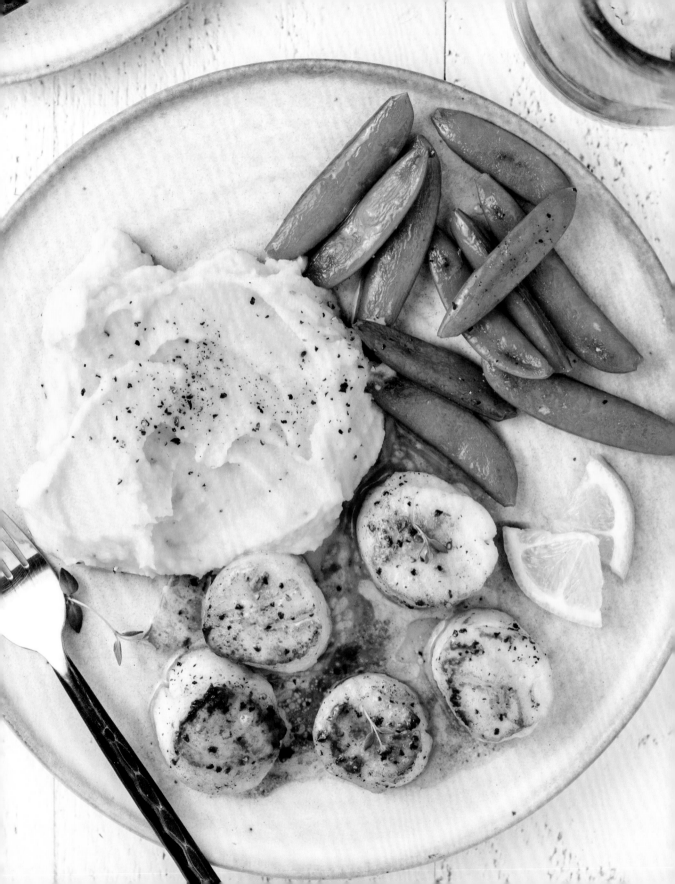

SEARED SCALLOPS IN BROWN BUTTER SAUCE

Scallops are a delicious and easy seafood dinner. They are a low-calorie, protein-rich option, high in magnesium and potassium. This simple preparation sears the scallops, then flavors them with a decadent herbed brown butter sauce. The amount of butter in this dish may seem like a lot, but if you use pastured butter, you'll benefit from its higher omega-3 content as well as conjugated linoleic acid (CLA) in high amounts, a nutrient that improves cardiovascular disease, cancer, chronic inflammation, and the immune system.

1 pound (454 g) sea scallops

1 tablespoon (15 ml) avocado oil

Sea salt and black pepper to taste

¼ cup (½ stick; 56 g) pastured butter, cut into pieces

4 fresh sage leaves

2 thyme sprigs

2 teaspoons fresh lemon juice

Pat the scallops dry with paper towels. This prevents the oil from splattering while browning the scallops.

In a large skillet over high heat, heat the oil. Add the scallops and season with salt and pepper to taste. Cook for about 4 minutes until the scallops caramelize on the bottom. Flip the scallops and add the butter and herbs to the skillet. Cook the scallops in the butter for 4 to 6 minutes, watching the butter as it begins to brown. Stop cooking when the butter has turned a deep golden-brown color.

Add the lemon juice and spoon the butter sauce over the scallops, flipping them a couple of times to coat in the flavors. Serve the scallops with a scoop of the butter sauce over the top.

YIELD

4 SERVINGS

NUTRITIONAL ANALYSIS

PER SERVING (ABOUT 5 SCALLOPS WITH ONE-FOURTH OF THE BROWN BUTTER SAUCE):

211 CALORIES

16G FAT

14G PROTEIN

4G CARBOHYDRATE

0G DIETARY FIBER

NOTE

This dish is perfect served with a veggie mash, such as my Cauliflower Parsnip Mash (page 121) and sautéed sugar snap peas. Drizzle the remaining brown butter over the mash—it's too good to waste.

COCONUT SHRIMP

Mix up your dinner routine with a dine-out favorite. This coconut shrimp sticks to the basics to keep it pegan. Don't be afraid to occasionally deep-fry. Because the shrimp are cooked at a high temperature, the cooking oil you use is especially important. I prefer the neutral taste of avocado oil, but use coconut oil if that is what you prefer.

Avocado oil, for frying

1 pound (454 g) shrimp, peeled and deveined

1 large egg

½ teaspoon sea salt

¼ teaspoon black pepper

1½ cups (128 g) unsweetened shredded coconut

In a large shallow skillet over medium-low heat, heat 1½ inches (3.5 cm) of oil until lightly golden brown. The exact amount of oil you'll need will depend on the size of your skillet.

Pat the shrimp dry with paper towels and set aside. Line a plate with paper towels and set aside.

In a small bowl, whisk the egg, salt, and pepper to blend. Place the coconut into a medium-size bowl.

One at a time, dip the shrimp in the egg, then the coconut, flipping to coat the shrimp heavily. Working in batches, carefully place the shrimp in the hot oil and fry for 30 to 45 seconds per side until the coconut is golden brown and the shrimp are fully cooked through. Transfer to the paper towel–lined plate to drain until ready to serve.

YIELD

4 SERVINGS

NUTRITIONAL ANALYSIS

PER SERVING (4 OUNCES, OR 115 G):

324 CALORIES

23G FAT

25G PROTEIN

3G CARBOHYDRATE

2G DIETARY FIBER

NOTE

The first few shrimp might not turn out perfectly. I start by cooking just one to test the temperature of the cooking oil, making sure the coconut browns and the shrimp are cooked through at the same time. If the shrimp are undercooked, turn down the heat so the shrimp can cook longer in the hot oil without burning or overbrowning the coconut.

ADD IT!

Try this fun shrimp served with a healthy dipping sauce. My Mango-Tarragon Dressing (page 154) is great choice. I like to add a few teaspoons of a paleo sriracha to the dressing to kick the heat up a notch. Beware of store-bought chili sauces that use sugar as a base.

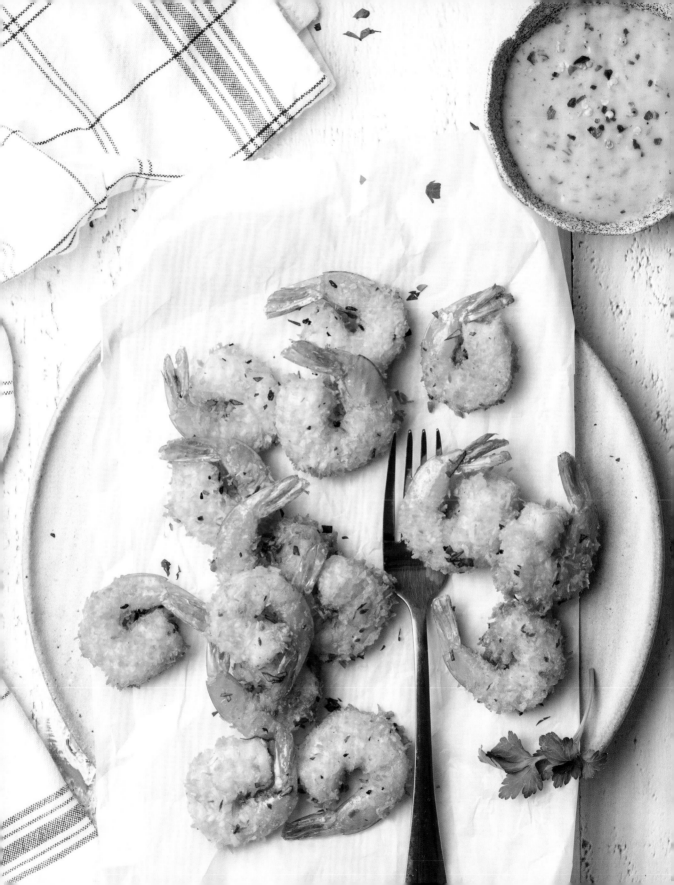

DON'T FEAR CIOPPINO

Seafood is incredibly nutritious, but people are often intimidated to cook it at home. Cioppino is my favorite Italian dish to eat out, but until recently, I felt it would be too difficult to make at home. That couldn't be further from the truth! This warming seafood stew is easy to make and is guaranteed to satisfy your seafood cravings.

¼ cup (60 ml) avocado oil

1 large fennel bulb, thinly sliced

1 onion, chopped

3 shallots, chopped

8 garlic cloves, finely chopped

1½ teaspoons sea salt, plus more for seasoning

¾ teaspoon red pepper flakes, plus more for seasoning

1½ cups (360 ml) dry white wine

1 (18-ounce, or 509 g) jar diced tomatoes

1 (32-ounce, or 908 ml) carton organic fish stock

2 bay leaves

1 pound (454 g) manila clams, scrubbed

1 pound (454 g) mussels, scrubbed and debearded

1 pound (454 g) raw large shrimp, peeled and deveined

1 pound (454 g) halibut or salmon, cut into 2-inch (5 cm) chunks

YIELD

8 SERVINGS

NUTRITIONAL ANALYSIS

PER SERVING (1½ CUPS, WEIGHT VARIES):

238 CALORIES

11G FAT

25G PROTEIN

9G CARBOHYDRATE

2G DIETARY FIBER

In a large Dutch oven over medium heat, heat the oil. Add the fennel, onion, shallots, and garlic. Sauté for about 10 minutes until the vegetables are softened. Season with the salt and red pepper flakes.

Add the white wine and simmer for 10 to 15 minutes until the wine is reduced by half.

Add the tomatoes, fish stock, and bay leaves. Simmer the stew for 20 minutes.

Add the clams and mussels to the pot, cover the pot, and cook for about 5 minutes until the clams and mussels begin to open.

Add the shrimp and halibut and cook for 5 minutes, uncovered. Discard any clams or mussels that have not opened.

Taste the stew and season with more salt and red pepper flakes, if necessary.

NOTE

Cioppino originates in San Francisco, not Italy, and is classically made with "seven seafoods." If you find purchasing seven different seafoods a stretch like I do, just use your favorites. This dish is easily made with just clams and shrimp, or only mussels and salmon. Experiment to find your favorite combinations.

ADD IT!

If you want to make this a special meal, by all means, add seven seafoods. Dungeness crab, squid, and scallops are great additions to this healthy stew.

TURKEY SWEET POTATO CHILI

A warming and filling meal year-round, this healthy turkey chili is a family favorite and a satisfying meal for active days.

1 tablespoon (15 ml) olive oil

1 onion, diced

3 garlic cloves, minced

2 pounds (908 g) pastured ground turkey

3 tablespoons (22 g) chili powder, plus more for seasoning (see note)

2 tablespoons (14 g) ground cumin

2 tablespoons (14 g) paprika

1 teaspoon dried oregano

1 teaspoon sea salt, plus more for seasoning

1 (28-ounce, or 794 g) jar diced tomatoes

1 (7-ounce, or 200 g) jar tomato paste

2 cups (480 ml) Anti-Inflammatory Chicken Bone Broth (page 137) or store-bought broth

1 pound (454 g) sweet potatoes, peeled and cut into 1-inch (2.5 cm) cubes

2 bell peppers, any color, cored and chopped

1 zucchini, chopped

YIELD

8 SERVINGS

NUTRITIONAL ANALYSIS

PER SERVING (1½ CUPS, OR ABOUT 300 G):

271 CALORIES

6G FAT

31G PROTEIN

28G CARBOHYDRATE

7G DIETARY FIBER

Heat a large soup pot or Dutch oven over medium heat. Pour in the oil and add the onion and garlic. Sauté for 5 to 7 minutes until softened.

Add the ground turkey and cook for 10 minutes, breaking it up into small pieces as it cooks and letting the turkey start to brown. While the turkey cooks, add the chili powder, cumin, paprika, oregano, and salt.

Stir in the diced tomatoes, tomato paste, chicken broth, sweet potatoes, and bell peppers. Simmer the chili for about 35 minutes until the sweet potatoes are soft and the chili has thickened.

Add the zucchini and simmer for 5 to 10 minutes more. Taste and adjust the seasonings and spice as needed.

NOTE

Chili powders vary greatly in heat and intensity, so be sure you know the strength of your chili powder before adding the full amount to this recipe. The chili powder I use is mild.

ADD IT!

Butternut squash is a great substitute for sweet potatoes, but it needs to be chopped and roasted first. To roast butternut squash, preheat the oven to 425°F (220°C, or gas mark 7). Place the peeled, chopped butternut squash cubes on a large sheet pan and spray with avocado oil. Roast the squash for about 20 minutes until softened, then add it to the chili with the zucchini.

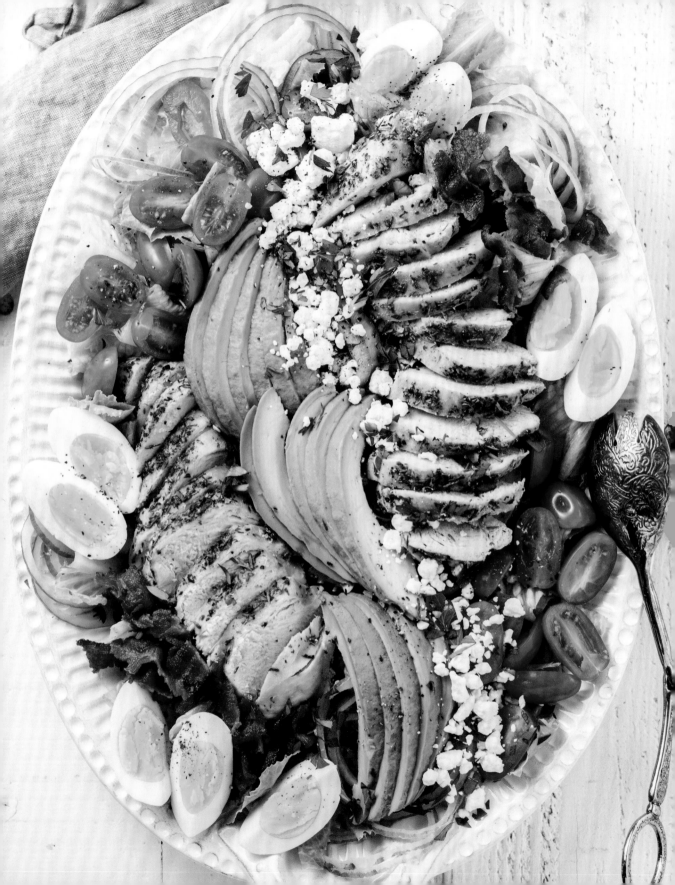

CLEANED-UP COBB SALAD

Making a few adjustments to a classic cobb salad turns a calorie-bomb meal into a nutrient-dense choice. This salad layers healthy proteins and fats with low-carb veggies.

FOR LEMON-THYME CHICKEN:

1 pound (454 g) organic chicken breasts

1 tablespoon (15 ml) olive oil

2 tablespoons (30 ml) fresh lemon juice

2 tablespoons (5 g) fresh thyme leaves, or 1½ teaspoons dried thyme

¾ teaspoon sea salt

Black pepper to taste

FOR COBB SALAD:

1 head romaine lettuce, chopped (about 6 cups, or 330 g)

6 nitrite- and nitrate-free bacon slices, cooked and crumbled

2 large eggs, hard-boiled, peeled, and quartered

1 large avocado, halved, peeled, pitted, and sliced

1 cup (149 g) cherry tomatoes, halved

½ cup (80 g) thinly sliced red onion

½ cup (75 g) goat cheese

¼ cup (120 ml) Balsamic Dijon Vinaigrette (page 148) or other favorite dressing

To make the lemon-thyme chicken: In a lidded container or large resealable plastic bag, combine the chicken, oil, lemon juice, and seasonings. Cover and gently shake to coat the chicken evenly with the seasonings. Refrigerate for at least 1 hour, and up to overnight.

Heat a skillet over medium heat. Remove the chicken from the marinade and add it to the skillet. Cook the chicken for 10 minutes per side, or until the chicken is cooked through and no longer pink. Let cool slightly and thinly slice the chicken. Discard the marinade.

To make the cobb salad: On a platter, arrange the romaine, bacon, eggs, avocado, tomatoes, red onion, and goat cheese. Add the chicken to the salad.

Serve the salad with the vinaigrette on the side.

YIELD

4 SERVINGS

NUTRITIONAL ANALYSIS*

PER SERVING (¼ RECIPE):

528 CALORIES

36G FAT

40G PROTEIN

14G CARBOHYDRATE

7G DIETARY FIBER

*NUTRITION FACTS DO NOT INCLUDE VINAIGRETTE

NOTE

Reduce the calories of this meal by using half the avocado and cheese or omitting one or both of these ingredients. The vinaigrette and bacon provide enough healthy fats to help your body access all the nutrients in the veggies.

TOM KHA GAI

Tom kha gai *translates to "chicken coconut milk soup." This version is infused with traditional flavors but has extra veggies to make it a complete and nourishing meal. This dish is traditionally served with steamed rice, but try quinoa or cauliflower rice for a change.*

1 tablespoon (15 ml) avocado oil

½ cup (50 g) sliced peeled fresh ginger

½ cup (80 g) sliced Thai shallots

3 (4-inch, or 10 cm) pieces lemongrass, cut into 1-inch (2.5 cm) pieces

4 cups (960 ml) Waste-Not Vegetable Broth (page 139) or store-bought broth

1 pound (454 g) pastured boneless, skinless chicken thighs, thinly sliced

1 carrot, diced

2 cups (130 g) sugar snap peas, ends trimmed, halved

2 cups (140 g) sliced mushrooms

2 (13.5-ounce, or 400 ml) cans full-fat coconut milk

4 Makrut lime leaves, or 1 tablespoon (6 g) grated lime zest

1 to 3 teaspoons (5 to 15 ml) paleo sriracha

Sea salt to taste

Lime wedges, for garnish

Chopped fresh cilantro, for garnish

In a large soup pot over medium heat, combine the oil, ginger, shallots, and lemongrass. Sauté for about 10 minutes to begin releasing the flavors.

Add the vegetable broth and chicken thighs and let simmer for about 5 minutes.

Add the carrot, sugar snap peas, and mushrooms, then stir in the coconut milk.

Tear the lime leaves to help release their oils and add them to the soup. Turn the heat to low and simmer the soup for about 10 minutes. Taste the soup and adjust the seasonings by adding sriracha and salt to taste.

Serve the soup by squeezing a lime wedge into each bowl and topping the soup with fresh cilantro.

YIELD

6 SERVINGS

NUTRITIONAL ANALYSIS

PER SERVING (1½ CUPS, OR 360 ML):

349 CALORIES

31G FAT

13G PROTEIN

11G CARBOHYDRATE

2G DIETARY FIBER

ADD IT!

Add chopped zucchini, broccoli, red bell pepper, asparagus, or even shredded cabbage, depending on what veggies you need to use.

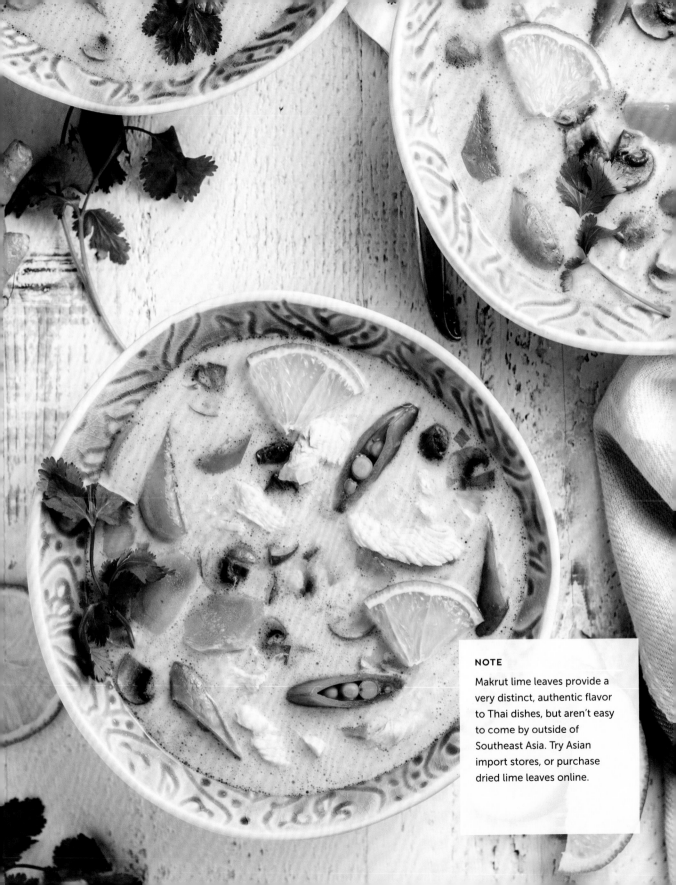

NOTE

Makrut lime leaves provide a very distinct, authentic flavor to Thai dishes, but aren't easy to come by outside of Southeast Asia. Try Asian import stores, or purchase dried lime leaves online.

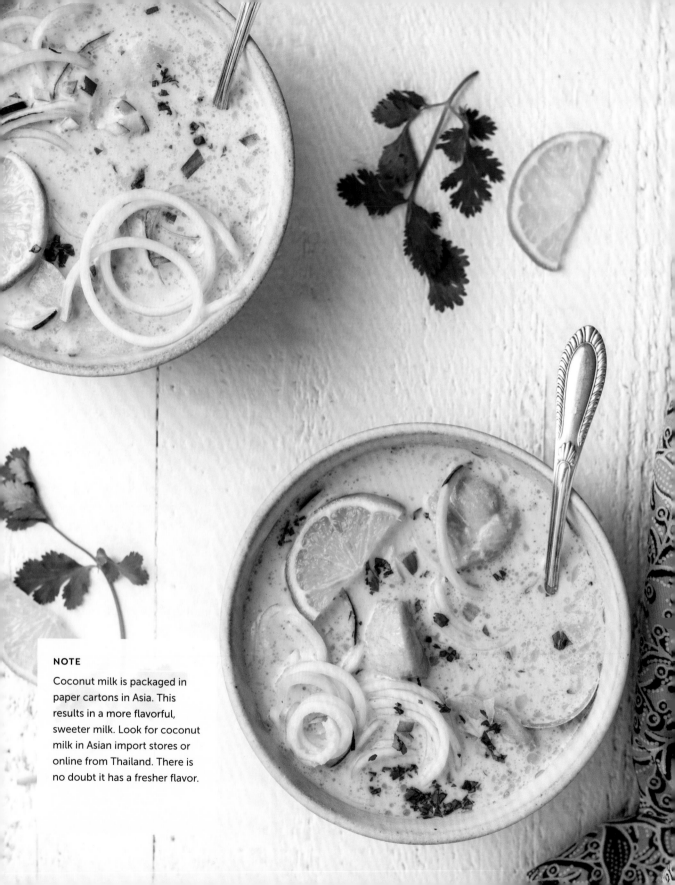

NOTE

Coconut milk is packaged in paper cartons in Asia. This results in a more flavorful, sweeter milk. Look for coconut milk in Asian import stores or online from Thailand. There is no doubt it has a fresher flavor.

IMMUNE-BOOSTING CHICKEN ZOODLE SOUP

Easy to make and bursting with nutrition, this soup amplifies the healing powers of chicken noodle soup. Ginger and turmeric both have powerful anti-inflammatory properties and coconut milk contains lauric acid, known to support the immune system. This soup comes together in about 30 minutes and is soul satisfying.

1 ounce (28 g) peeled fresh ginger

1 tablespoon (15 ml) avocado oil

1 teaspoon ground turmeric

2 pounds (908 g) pastured boneless chicken, cut into 1-inch (2.5 cm) chunks

3 cups (720 ml) Anti-Inflammatory Chicken Bone Broth (page 137) or store-bought broth

1 cup (160 g) chopped red onion

1 (13-ounce, or 375 ml) can full-fat coconut milk

3 tablespoons (45 ml) coconut aminos

1 tablespoon (20 g) maple syrup (optional)

1 tablespoon (15 ml) fresh lime juice

1 to 3 teaspoons (5 to 15 ml) paleo sriracha, plus more for seasoning

Sea salt to taste

2 or 3 zucchini, spiralized

Chopped fresh cilantro, for garnish

Lime wedges, for serving

Use a sharp knife to cut the ginger into very thin slices. The thinner the slices, the less sharp/pungent the flavor will be in the soup.

In a large soup pot over medium heat, combine the oil, ginger slices, and turmeric. Sauté for about 5 minutes to soften.

Add the chicken, chicken broth, and red onion. Simmer the soup for about 20 minutes to cook the chicken fully.

Stir in the coconut milk, coconut aminos, maple syrup (if using), lime juice, and sriracha. Taste and adjust the seasonings by adding salt to taste (depending on whether your chicken broth has salt) or more sriracha for spiciness.

To serve, place 1 cup (120 g) raw zucchini noodles into each serving bowl and ladle the hot soup on top. This keeps the zucchini noodles from overcooking and becoming mushy in the soup pot. Sprinkle with cilantro and serve with a lime wedge.

Refrigerate leftover zucchini noodles and the soup separately for up to 3 days. To serve, reheat the soup and serve on top of the raw zucchini noodles.

YIELD

8 SERVINGS

NUTRITIONAL ANALYSIS

PER SERVING (1 CUP, OR 120 G, ZUCCHINI NOODLES AND 1 CUP, OR 240 ML, SOUP):

411 CALORIES

32G FAT

21G PROTEIN

10G CARBOHYDRATE

1G DIETARY FIBER

ADD IT!

If you don't have a spiralizer, use a vegetable peeler to shave the zucchini into long strands. Move the peeler around the outside of the zucchini, end to end, until you hit the core. Freeze the core to toss into smoothies.

CREAMY SAUSAGE, CELERIAC, AND KALE SOUP

A winter night's dream. This healthy "cream" soup is made with a nutritious blend of cashews and cauliflower. The soup gets most of its flavor from the sausage, so buy a brand that you really enjoy. Rather than potatoes, this soup uses a lower-carb, lesser-known vegetable, celeriac. Celeriac softens as it cooks and gets a creamy texture and has a mild, sweet flavor.

½ cup (70 g) cashews, soaked in water overnight

6 cups (600 g) roughly chopped cauliflower

¾ cup (180 ml) water

1 tablespoon (15 ml) olive oil

1 onion, chopped

3 garlic cloves, minced

1 pound (454 g) pastured pork Italian sausage

6 cups (1.4 L) Anti-Inflammatory Chicken Bone Broth (page 137) or store-bought broth

1 large celeriac (celery root), peeled and cut into 1-inch (2.5 cm) cubes

1 bunch lacinato kale, chopped

½ teaspoon dried basil

½ teaspoon dried thyme

¼ to ½ teaspoon red pepper flakes

Sea salt and black pepper to taste

YIELD

6 SERVINGS

NUTRITIONAL ANALYSIS

PER SERVING (2 CUPS, OR 480 ML):

451 CALORIES

28G FAT

24G PROTEIN

28G CARBOHYDRATE

3G DIETARY FIBER

Drain and rinse the cashews. Set aside.

Place a steamer basket in a large pot and add 1 inch (2.5 cm) of water to the pot. Place the pot over medium-high heat. Place the cauliflower in the basket, cover, and steam for 15 minutes, or until very soft. Drain and transfer to a blender.

Add the cashews and water. Process for 2 to 3 minutes until a smooth cream forms. Set aside.

Heat a large soup pot over medium heat. Pour in the oil and add the onion and garlic. Cook for about 10 minutes to soften, being careful not to brown the onion and garlic. The soup will be silky white if the onions aren't overbrowned.

Add the sausage to the pot and cook for about 10 minutes until it begins to brown.

Add the chicken broth and celeriac. Cook for 15 minutes so the celeriac softens.

Stir in the cauliflower cream sauce, kale, and seasonings. Simmer for 5 to 10 minutes more, tasting and adjusting the seasonings based on your preference and how flavorful the sausage is.

NOTE

As with other cuts of meats, buy humanely raised pastured pork sausage. If you'd like to lighten up this dish, make it with an organic chicken sausage.

NOTE

Soups are great for freezing. Serve portions of this soup with Garlic and Rosemary Almond Meal Flaxseed Crackers (page 40) for easy meals during busy weeks.

SESAME-GINGER GRILLED CHICKEN

This simple marinade takes minutes to put together and results in perfectly moist and flavorful chicken every time. Any chicken (boneless, white, or dark meat) works with this marinade, but you'll reap the benefits of the connective tissues if you choose bone-in thighs, wings, and drumsticks. Creamy Asian-Style Cucumber Noodles (page 128) are the perfect pairing for this dish.

2 pounds (908 g) bone-in pastured chicken pieces

1 cup (240 ml) coconut aminos

3 tablespoons (45 ml) toasted sesame oil

1 tablespoon (6 g) ground ginger

1 teaspoon sea salt

1 tablespoon (15 ml) paleo sriracha (optional)

Place the chicken in a large lidded container and add the coconut aminos, sesame oil, ginger, salt, and sriracha (if using). Place the lid on the container and gently shake to mix the ingredients and coat the chicken evenly. Refrigerate the chicken for at least 5 hours, and up to overnight.

Preheat a grill or a grill pan to medium heat. Place the marinated chicken on the grill and cook for about 10 minutes per side until the internal temperature reaches 165°F (74°C). Larger pieces of chicken will need to cook longer. Use a meat thermometer to check the internal temperature.

YIELD

4 SERVINGS

NUTRITIONAL ANALYSIS (USING BONE-IN CHICKEN THIGHS)

PER SERVING (8 OUNCES, OR 225 G):

577 CALORIES

43G FAT

37G PROTEIN

7G CARBOHYDRATE

1G DIETARY FIBER

NOTE

Boneless chicken thighs marinate more quickly than bone-in pieces. If making a substitution, reduce the marinating time to about 4 hours.

NOTE

I use this marinade often, so I keep it super simple to throw together, but if you have a few more minutes, using fresh ginger in this recipe is a delicious option. Grate ¼ cup (32 g) peeled fresh ginger and add it to the marinade in place of the ground ginger.

ROASTED TURKEY LEGS
WITH VEGETABLES

Turkey legs are a great protein option. Meats with a lot of connective tissue and joints are higher in fat and collagen, nutrients that improve joint health, skin elasticity, and wound healing. This delicious part of the turkey is quick and easy to roast with vegetables for a satisfying, nutritious meal.

6 pastured turkey legs

Sea salt and black pepper to taste

2 tablespoons (28 g) pastured butter, at room temperature

2 tablespoons (5 g) chopped fresh sage

2 teaspoons poultry seasoning

2 apples, quartered and cored

1 onion, quartered

12 Brussels sprouts, halved

½ cup (120 ml) Anti-Inflammatory Chicken Bone Broth (page 137) or store-bough broth

Preheat the oven to 350°F (180°C, or gas mark 4).

Place the turkey legs in a large baking dish and generously season with salt and pepper.

In a small bowl, stir together the butter, sage, and poultry seasoning. Use a spoon to blend the spices into the butter. Using your hands, rub each turkey leg with some of the herbed butter.

Add the apples, onion, and Brussels sprouts to the baking dish around the turkey legs. Pour the chicken broth into the dish.

Bake for 1 hour, 30 minutes, or until the turkey legs reach an internal temperature of 170°F (77°C) measured on a meat thermometer.

Drain the drippings from the pan into a saucepan and prepare Apple-Sage Turkey Gravy (page 136), if desired, to serve.

YIELD

6 SERVINGS

NUTRITIONAL ANALYSIS

PER SERVING (1 [11-OUNCE, OR 308 G] TURKEY LEG, ⅔ CUP, OR ABOUT 120 G, ROASTED APPLES AND VEGETABLES):

470 CALORIES

23G FAT

53G PROTEIN

14G CARBOHYDRATE

3G DIETARY FIBER

NOTE

Turn this dish into a holiday-worthy meal by serving it with Cauliflower Parsnip Mash (page 121) and Apple-Sage Turkey Gravy (page 136). This is a great recipe for a holiday meal for two or three people, when a whole turkey isn't necessary.

ADD IT!

A variety of vegetables works well in this dish, including carrots, sweet potatoes, parsnips, turnips, and cauliflower. Simply replace any of the vegetables or the apples in the dish with your choice.

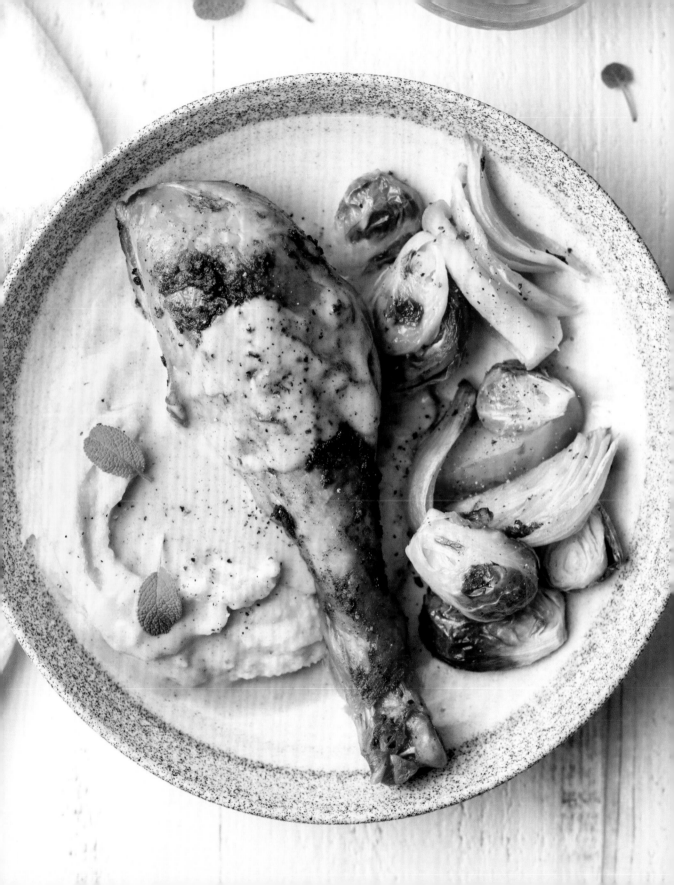

MAPLE-DIJON PORK TENDERLOIN WITH WATERCRESS AND APPLE SALAD

This recipe will soon become a favorite for family gatherings or entertaining. The presentation is gorgeous and yet it takes less than 30 minutes from start to finish to put together. Fresh, crisp apple, fennel, and watercress salad adds crunch and puts a lively spin on the classic pork roast and applesauce.

**FOR MAPLE-DIJON
PORK TENDERLOIN:**

1 tablespoon (15 ml) avocado oil

2 pounds (908 g) pastured pork
   tenderloins

Sea salt and black pepper to taste

3 tablespoons (45 g) Dijon mustard

2 tablespoons (40 g) maple syrup

1 tablespoon (10 g) crushed garlic

2 tablespoons (5 g) fresh
   thyme leaves

**FOR WATERCRESS
AND APPLE SALAD:**

2 fennel bulbs

2 tart apples

½ cup (120 ml) fresh lemon juice

6 tablespoons (90 ml) balsamic
   vinegar

6 tablespoons (90 ml) olive oil

6 cups (330 g) watercress,
   stems trimmed

Sea salt and black pepper to taste

To make the maple-Dijon pork tenderloin: Preheat the oven to 450°F (230°C, or gas mark 8).

In a cast-iron skillet over high heat, heat the oil. Add the pork tenderloins and generously season with salt and pepper to taste. Cook for 2 to 3 minutes per side to lightly brown, then remove from the heat.

In a small bowl, whisk the Dijon, maple syrup, garlic, and thyme to combine. Drizzle two-thirds of the mixture over the pork, evenly coating the meat.

Move the skillet to the oven and roast for 15 to 20 minutes, or until the pork reaches an internal temperature of 140°F to 155°F (60°C to 70°C), basting with the remaining sauce about halfway through the cooking time. The temperature for medium-rare meat is 145°F (63°C), but the meat will continue cooking after it's removed from the oven, so it's best to take it out before the desired temperature is reached.

Let the pork rest for at least 5 minutes before slicing and serving.

To make the watercress and apple salad: While the pork cooks, prepare the salad. Thinly slice the fennel bulbs and place in a large bowl. I like to do this with a mandoline so the slices are thin and crunchy, rather than chewy. Very thinly slice the apples and mix with the fennel. Drizzle the apples and fennel with the lemon juice, vinegar, and oil and toss to coat.

Place the watercress on a serving platter and top with the apple and fennel mixture. Season with salt and pepper to taste. Add the sliced pork tenderloin to the platter to serve.

8 SERVINGS

NUTRITIONAL ANALYSIS

PER SERVING (4 OUNCES, OR 115 G,
PORK PLUS 1 CUP, WEIGHT VARIES,
WATERCRESS AND APPLE SALAD):

287 CALORIES

13G FAT

25G PROTEIN

17G CARBOHYDRATE

3G DIETARY FIBER

NOTE

Purchase heritage or pastured
pork products to ensure the
animal was raised humanely
and was allowed to forage for
a natural diet of fruit, grubs,
and acorns. Conventionally
raised pigs are fed a diet of
GMO soy, corn, and wheat,
which is not ideal for the
health of the animal or our
environment, and it degrades
the nutrition of the meat.

ADD IT!

This dish makes a delicious
light meal on its own. It also
pairs wonderfully with the
earthy sweetness of Cauliflower
Parsnip Mash (page 121) and
Crispy Roasted Brussels Sprouts
and Radishes (page 120).

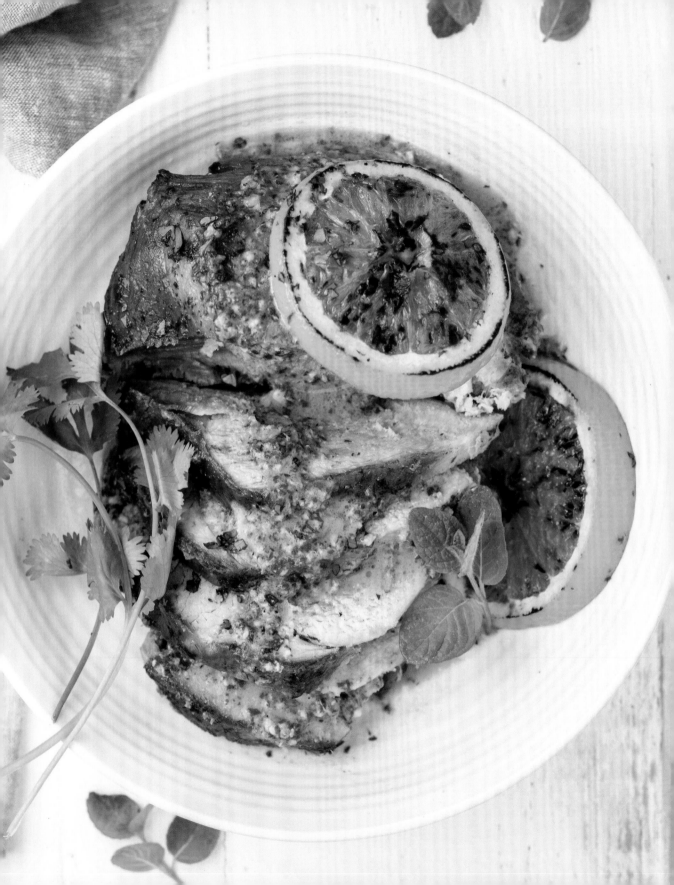

MOJO PORK ROAST

My absolute favorite way to enjoy pork is this mojo pork roast. This Cuban-inspired recipe combines bright citrus, mint, cilantro, and garlic for a tender roast bursting with flavor. The marinade takes minutes to prepare, but this recipe is best if you allow a full 24 hours of marinating time. The roast is slow cooked for more than 2 hours, so although the process is mostly hands off, be sure to plan ahead.

1 (2-pound, or 908 g) pastured pork sirloin roast

½ cup (120 ml) fresh orange juice

½ cup (8 g) tightly packed fresh cilantro

⅓ cup (80 ml) fresh lime juice

¼ cup (24 g) tightly packed fresh mint leaves

3 tablespoons (45 ml) avocado oil

4 garlic cloves, peeled

1 teaspoon ground cumin

1 teaspoon sea salt

½ teaspoon black pepper

Place the pork roast in a lidded storage container.

In a blender, combine the remaining ingredients and process until the garlic and herbs are well chopped but there is still some texture to the marinade. Pour the marinade over the pork and refrigerate to marinate for at least 4 hours, but marinating for 24 hours yields the most flavorful and tender roast.

Preheat the oven to 300°F (150°C, or gas mark 2).

Transfer the pork roast to a baking pan with a rack and tightly wrap the pan with aluminum foil, tenting the foil to prevent it from sticking to the roast. Reserve the marinade.

Bake for 2½ hours. Remove the foil and increase the oven temperature to 425°F (220°C, or gas mark 7). Bake for 30 minutes more to brown the roast, or until the internal temperature reaches 160°F (70°C). Let rest for 10 minutes before carving.

When the roast is nearly done, place the marinade in a small saucepan over medium-low heat and simmer until it's reduced by half.

Carve the roast into thick slices and serve drizzled with the reduced marinade.

YIELD

8 SERVINGS

NUTRITIONAL ANALYSIS

PER SERVING (4 OUNCES, OR 115 G):

187 CALORIES

7G FAT

26G PROTEIN

3G CARBOHYDRATE

1G DIETARY FIBER

NOTE

Serve this moist, tender pork roast with cauliflower rice, zucchini noodles, or even use it in place of the ground beef on the Kale Taco Salad (page 111). I love this recipe served with lettuce wraps, avocado, and a spicy salsa. However you choose to serve it, add plenty of veggies to your plate.

VIETNAMESE-STYLE PORK BÁNH MÌ BOWLS

This is a fun twist on the popular Southeast Asian sandwich, the bánh mì. The keys to its deliciousness are the pickled vegetables and spicy mayo. This pegan version uses a base of cucumber noodles and spiralized carrot and daikon radish to make it similar to a cold noodle dish. I've been making these with pork tenderloin, but chicken thighs are a great substitute.

FOR PORK TENDERLOIN:

1 (1-pound, or 454 g) pastured pork tenderloin

3 tablespoons (45 ml) coconut aminos

3 tablespoons (45 ml) rice wine vinegar

1 tablespoon (15 g) tahini

1 tablespoon (20 g) maple syrup

½ teaspoon sea salt

FOR BÁNH MÌ BOWLS:

6 tablespoons (90 ml) rice wine vinegar

2 tablespoons (30 ml) sesame oil

1 tablespoon (20 g) maple syrup

1 teaspoon sea salt

1 pound (454 g) daikon radishes, spiralized

2 large carrots, spiralized

2 English cucumbers, spiralized

¼ cup (56 g) avocado oil mayonnaise

1 to 3 teaspoons (5 to 15 ml) paleo sriracha

¼ cup (4 g) chopped fresh cilantro

To make the pork tenderloin: Thinly slice the pork tenderloin. This is easiest to do if the pork is partially frozen. If your tenderloin is fully thawed, place it in the freezer for 20 minutes before slicing.

In a large lidded container, stir together the coconut aminos, vinegar, tahini, maple syrup, and salt. Add the sliced pork and toss it to fully coat. Cover and refrigerate the pork while preparing the other ingredients.

In a large skillet over high heat, cook the pork for 7 to 10 minutes, flipping frequently to cook it evenly until it reaches an internal temperature of 145°F (63°C). Discard the marinade.

To make the bánh mì bowls: In a large lidded storage container, combine the vinegar, oil, maple syrup, and salt. Cover and shake to combine. Add the daikon radishes and carrots to the container. Re-cover and shake to coat the vegetables evenly.

Into each of 4 bowls, place one-fourth of the spiralized cucumber and one-fourth of the daikon radish and carrot mixture.

In a small dish, stir together the mayonnaise and sriracha.

Top each vegetable noodle bowl with pork, 1 tablespoon (1 g) of cilantro, and a drizzle of sriracha mayo.

YIELD

4 SERVINGS

NUTRITIONAL ANALYSIS

PER SERVING (4 OUNCES, OR 115 G, PORK, 2 CUPS, WEIGHT VARIES, SPIRALIZED VEGGIES, AND 1 TABLESPOON, OR 14 G, SRIRACHA MAYO):

354 CALORIES

16G FAT

26G PROTEIN

24G CARBOHYDRATE

4G DIETARY FIBER

NOTE

If you don't have a spiralizer, halve the vegetables lengthwise, then very thinly slice them. A spiralizer is one of my favorite kitchen gadgets—it turns salads into dishes that feel more like noodles. I recommend investing in one.

NOTE

If you're eating a lower-carb diet or are diabetic and need to lower the carbs in this dish, replace the maple syrup with a monk fruit– or stevia-based sweetener to taste.

GRILLED ROSEMARY PORK SKEWERS

Up your grilling game with a flavorful marinade. If you love to grill in summer, these pork skewers will become a new favorite. The char that results from high-heat grilling produces heterocyclic amines, a carcinogen, but marinating meats reduces the amount produced. I love cutting the meat, marinating it, and then skewering it for maximum flavor, but you can also use this marinade on whole chops to save time.

2 pounds (908 g) boneless pastured pork loin chops, cut into 1-inch (2.5 cm) cubes

¼ cup (60 ml) balsamic vinegar

¼ cup (7 g) finely chopped fresh rosemary leaves

2 tablespoons (30 ml) avocado oil

2 tablespoons (30 ml) fresh lemon juice

1 tablespoon (15 g) Dijon mustard

4 garlic cloves, minced

2 teaspoons sea salt

Black pepper to taste

Place the pork in an airtight container.

In a small bowl, whisk the vinegar, rosemary, oil, lemon juice, Dijon, garlic, salt, and pepper to combine. Pour the marinade over the pork. Use a fork to mix the marinade into the pork, coating it well. Cover the container and refrigerate to marinate for at least 2 hours, and up to overnight. The pork is especially flavorful if you have time to marinate overnight.

Once or twice during the marinating time, stir the pork in the marinade.

Preheat a grill to medium heat.

Divide the pork cubes among 8 skewers. Grill the pork skewers for 6 to 8 minutes per side until the outsides are lightly charred and the pork is cooked through to an internal temperature of 145°F (63°C). I prefer pork slightly pink in the center.

Alternatively, to cook these indoors, coat a grill pan with avocado oil and heat it over medium heat. Add the skewers and cook for 5 to 7 minutes per side, or until the pork looks evenly cooked though and reaches an internal temperature of 145°F (63°C).

YIELD

8 SKEWERS

NUTRITIONAL ANALYSIS

PER SERVING (1 SKEWER):

219 CALORIES

12G FAT

25G PROTEIN

3G CARBOHYDRATE

1G DIETARY FIBER

NOTE

This recipe works well with chicken and beef, too, so if you're having a cookout, remember to plan ahead and marinate the meat for the healthiest outcome.

ADD IT!

When hosting summer cookouts, I like to have most of the work done ahead, so I prepare easy salads and plan to cook the meats or some simple grilled veggies at mealtime. If you'd like to add some salads to round out this meal, try the Heirloom Tomato and Herb Salad (page 72) or the Summer Greek Salad (page 66), both of which are great prepped ahead. Remember to fill 75 percent of your plate with healthy veggies.

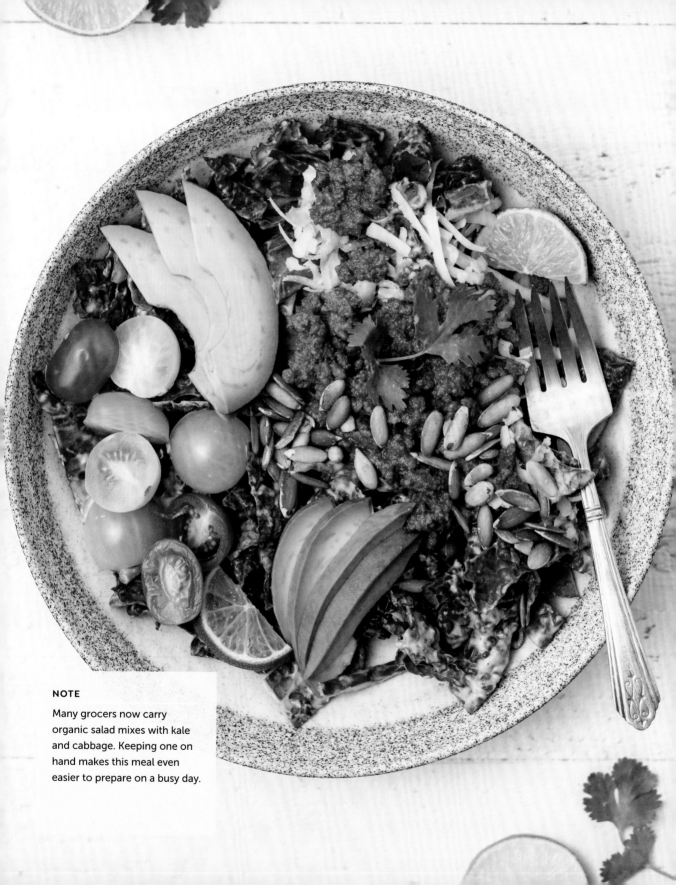

NOTE

Many grocers now carry organic salad mixes with kale and cabbage. Keeping one on hand makes this meal even easier to prepare on a busy day.

KALE TACO SALAD

Upgrade your taco salad with flavorful, nutrient-dense kale and a homemade grass-fed beef taco meat.

FOR KALE TACO SALAD:

6 cups (402 g) chopped lacinato kale

2 cups (140 g) shredded red cabbage

½ cup (120 ml) Spicy Avocado-Cilantro Dressing (page 149)

1 cup (150 g) cherry tomatoes, halved

½ avocado, peeled, pitted, and cut into chunks

½ cup (64 g) toasted pumpkin seeds

½ cup (130 g) salsa

½ cup (58 g) shredded raw Cheddar cheese (optional)

FOR TACO MEAT:

1 tablespoon (15 ml) avocado oil

1 pound (454 g) grass-fed ground beef

¼ cup (60 ml) Rosemary Beef Bone Broth (page 138) or store-bought beef broth or chicken broth

2 tablespoons (32 g) tomato paste

1 tablespoon (7 g) ground cumin

1 tablespoon (8 g) paprika

1½ teaspoons chili powder

1½ teaspoons garlic powder

1½ teaspoons onion powder

1 teaspoon sea salt, or to taste

To make the kale taco salad: In a large salad bowl, combine the kale, red cabbage, and dressing. Use your hands to massage the dressing into the vegetables. If you don't have time to make the dressing, see the note following. Cover the bowl and refrigerate while preparing the rest of the salad and taco meat.

To make the taco meat: In a large skillet over medium-high heat, heat the oil. Add the ground beef and cook for about 10 minutes, using a spatula to break up the meat as it browns.

Stir in the beef broth, tomato paste, and seasonings. Bring the taco meat to a simmer and cook until no liquid remains, stirring occasionally to cook the meat evenly.

To assemble the salad: When ready to serve, divide the kale mixture onto plates, top with the cherry tomatoes, avocado, pumpkin seeds, salsa, Cheddar cheese (if using), and taco meat.

YIELD

4 SERVINGS

NUTRITIONAL ANALYSIS*

PER SERVING (2 CUPS TACO SALAD, WEIGHT VARIES, PLUS 4 OUNCES, OR 115 G, TACO MEAT):

408 CALORIES

20G FAT

38G PROTEIN

24G CARBOHYDRATE

6G DIETARY FIBER

*NUTRITION FACTS DO NOT INCLUDE SALAD DRESSING

NOTE

Rather than prepare the Spicy Avocado-Cilantro Dressing, massage the kale and cabbage with 2 tablespoons (30 ml) avocado oil, 2 tablespoons (30 ml) fresh lime juice, and 2 tablespoons (30 ml) red or white wine vinegar, then season with a little salt and cumin. Massage the blend into the kale and allow it to soak in the dressing while preparing the taco meat.

SHEPHERD'S PIE WITH CAULIFLOWER PARSNIP CRUST

Lamb raised in the United States is most often grass fed. Meat raised on grass is higher in omega-3s and is a great source of protein and iron. This classic English dish is lightened up with a delicious earthy and slightly sweet cauliflower and parsnip crust. I use snap peas rather than shelled peas to add extra fiber and make the dish less starchy.

FOR CAULIFLOWER-PARSNIP TOPPING:

1 head (about 2 pounds, or 908 g) cauliflower, roughly chopped

2 parsnips, ends trimmed, sliced

1 tablespoon (14 g) pastured butter

Sea salt and black pepper to taste

FOR LAMB STEW:

1 tablespoon (15 ml) olive oil

1 small onion, minced

2 garlic cloves, minced

1 tablespoon (2 g) fresh rosemary leaves, chopped

1 teaspoon sea salt

Black pepper to taste

1 pound (454 g) ground grass-fed lamb

1 pound (454 g) mushrooms, chopped

3 carrots, sliced

1½ cups (100 g) sugar snap peas, ends trimmed, sliced

1 cup (240 ml) organic beef stock

2 tablespoons (30 ml) coconut aminos

2 tablespoons (32 g) tomato paste

2 tablespoons (16 g) arrowroot

2 tablespoons (30 ml) water

To make the cauliflower parsnip topping: Place a steamer basket in a large pot and add 1 inch (2.5 cm) of water to the pot. Place the pot over medium-high heat. Place the cauliflower and parsnips in the steamer basket, cover, and steam for 15 to 20 minutes until very tender. Drain and transfer the cauliflower and parsnips to a food processor. Add the butter, and salt and pepper to taste. Process until thick and smooth.

To make the lamb stew: Meanwhile, in a large skillet over medium heat, heat the oil. Add the onion and garlic and sauté for 5 to 7 minutes to soften. Add the rosemary and the salt and pepper.

Preheat the oven to 400°F (200°C, or gas mark 6).

Add the ground lamb to the skillet with the onion and garlic. Cook for 7 to 10 minutes, using a spatula to break up the meat as it browns.

Stir in the mushrooms, carrots, peas, beef stock, coconut aminos, and tomato paste. Bring to a simmer.

In a small dish, whisk the arrowroot and water to combine. Stir this slurry into the broth and simmer for 2 to 3 minutes to thicken. Pour the lamb mixture into a 9 × 9-inch (23 × 23 cm) baking dish. Scoop the cauliflower and parsnip mash over the top, dropping evenly spaced mounds around the top. Use a spatula or spoon to smooth the top.

Bake the casserole for 20 minutes, or until the top has lightly browned and the lamb mixture is bubbling.

ADD IT!

Add chopped broccoli, kale, or zucchini for more greens in your meal.

NUTRITIONAL ANALYSIS

PER SERVING:

387 CALORIES

23G FAT

20G PROTEIN

28G CARBOHYDRATE

7G DIETARY FIBER

NOTE

Modern versions of shepherd's pie use ground beef. Check for the American Grass Fed Association label to ensure your lamb was raised humanely and given access to a natural diet.

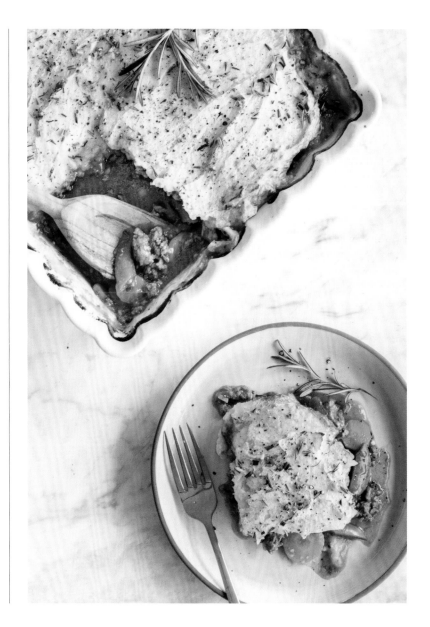

SEARED LAMB CHOPS
WITH CITRUS MINT SALAD

*Lamb is a highly nutritious meat, often overlooked. Most often lamb is grass fed,
so it's easy to know you are getting a high-quality meat. This recipe uses a simple
light marinade and pairs the lamb with a vibrant citrus mint salad.*

FOR SEARED LAMB CHOPS:

2 tablespoons (30 ml) avocado oil

2 tablespoons (30 ml) fresh
  lemon juice

4 garlic cloves, minced

1½ teaspoons sea salt

1 teaspoon paprika

1 teaspoon dried oregano

Black pepper to taste

2 pounds (908 g) bone-in
  grass-fed lamb chops

FOR CITRUS MINT SALAD:

1 blood orange, peeled and sliced
  crosswise

3 tangerines, peeled and sliced
  crosswise

2 tablespoons (12 g) chopped
  fresh mint

2 tablespoons (20 g) minced
  shallot

2 tablespoons (30 ml) avocado oil

1 tablespoon (15 ml) fresh
  lemon juice

1 tablespoon (20 g) honey

To make the lamb chops: In a small bowl, whisk the oil, lemon juice, garlic, salt, paprika, oregano, and pepper to taste to combine.

Put the lamb chops on a plate and drizzle the marinade over the top. Cover the dish and refrigerate to marinate for at least 30 minutes, and up to overnight, flipping the chops halfway through the marinating time.

To make the citrus mint salad: While the lamb marinates, arrange the citrus on a serving dish and sprinkle with the mint and shallot.

In a small bowl, whisk the oil, lemon juice, and honey to blend. Drizzle the dressing over the salad. Set aside.

To finish the dish: Heat a large skillet over medium-high heat. Add the lamb chops to the hot skillet, leaving some space between them. Cook for 3 to 4 minutes per side, based on your preferred doneness. Three minutes per side will result in lamb that is a medium doneness.

Serve the lamb chops drizzled with any pan drippings and serve the citrus mint salad on the side.

YIELD

4 SERVINGS

NUTRITIONAL ANALYSIS

PER SERVING (ABOUT 8 OUNCES, OR 225 G, LAMB CHOPS AND ⅓ CUP, WEIGHT VARIES, SALAD):

560 CALORIES

30G FAT

57G PROTEIN

14G CARBOHYDRATE

2G DIETARY FIBER

NOTE

This dish is delicious served with simple sides, like Sautéed Beet Greens (page 134) or Crispy Roasted Brussels Sprouts and Radishes (page 120).

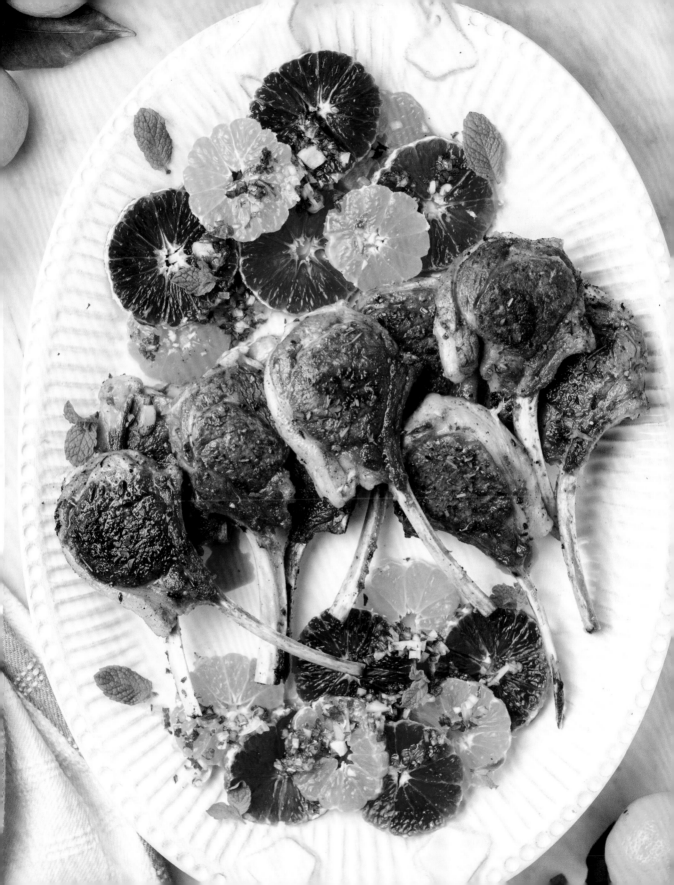

BEEF RENDANG

A popular dish in parts of Southeast Asia, this flavorful beef curry is unique and irresistible. Don't let the long ingredient list scare you—most items are easy to keep in the pantry and the dish comes together quickly and simmers into tender chunks of beef that fall apart in the sweet and spicy sauce. My family loves this served over cauliflower rice, but quinoa and a side of green veggies are just as good.

FOR MALAYSIAN STEWED BEEF:

2 tablespoons (30 ml) avocado oil

2 shallots, finely minced

3 stalks lemongrass, white parts only, tough outer layer removed, minced

2 inches (5 cm) fresh ginger, peeled and grated

1½ pounds (681 g) grass-fed beef stew meat

1 cinnamon stick

3 whole cloves

4 star anise

3 cardamom pods, smashed

6 Makrut lime leaves

1 (13.5-ounce, or 400 ml) can coconut cream

1 cup (240 ml) water

2 tablespoons (30 ml) fresh lime juice

¼ cup (21 g) toasted unsweetened coconut

1 tablespoon (15 g) coconut sugar

1 teaspoon sea salt, or to taste

Chopped fresh cilantro, for garnish (optional)

FOR CAULIFLOWER RICE:

1 tablespoon (15 ml) avocado oil

9 cups (900 g) riced cauliflower

Sea salt and black pepper to taste

To make the Malaysian stewed beef: In a Dutch oven over medium heat, combine the oil, shallots, lemongrass, and ginger. Stir-fry for 7 to 10 minutes until the ingredients are fragrant.

Add the stew meat, cinnamon stick, cloves, star anise, and cardamom pods. Stir-fry for 5 to 10 minutes to lightly brown the meat.

Add the lime leaves, coconut cream, water, lime juice, coconut, coconut sugar, and salt. Stir-fry to combine, then turn the heat to medium-low. Cover the pot and let the beef stew for 2 hours, stirring occasionally and ensuring there is enough water in the pot to continue simmering. If the liquid is getting low, add water, ¼ cup (60 ml) at a time, to rehydrate it while it continues to stew.

The beef is done when the sauce has thickened and is no longer a creamy color from the coconut cream.

To make the cauliflower rice: In a large skillet over high heat, heat the oil. Add the cauliflower rice and stir-fry for 5 to 6 minutes until heated throughout. Remove from the heat and season with salt and pepper to taste.

Serve the beef over the cauliflower rice garnished with cilantro (if using).

YIELD

6 SERVINGS

NUTRITIONAL ANALYSIS

PER SERVING (4 OUNCES, OR
115 G BEEF STEW, AND 1½ CUPS,
OR 160 G, CAULIFLOWER RICE):

656 CALORIES

54G FAT

27G PROTEIN

23G CARBOHYDRATE

7G DIETARY FIBER

NOTE

Fresh Makrut lime leaves are difficult to purchase outside of Asia but can be found dried from online retailers or at Asian import stores. They have a unique flavor that lends an authentic taste to Southeast Asian dishes. If you cannot find them, use 1 tablespoon (6 g) of grated lime zest instead.

NOTE

This dish is best when the beef is slowly cooked for a long time. The creamy color of the coconut cream will disappear, creating a thick and flavorful sauce.

GRASS-FED ROAST BEEF

Roast beef is simple to prepare and the thick slices of beef are a great option for serving over roasted vegetables, salads, or as a topper to Garlic and Rosemary Almond Meal Flaxseed Crackers (page 40). This garlic and herb-rubbed roast is prepared with vegetables for a one-pan meal. Leftover beef roast can be vacuum-sealed and frozen for easy protein to add to meals later.

1 (3-pound, or 1.4 kg) grass-fed beef chuck roast

2 tablespoons (30 ml) olive oil

2 tablespoons (3 g) chopped fresh rosemary leaves

4 garlic cloves, minced

1 tablespoon (2 g) fresh thyme leaves

1½ teaspoons sea salt

Black pepper to taste

1 pound (454 g) carrots, cut into chunks

2 large onions, quartered

2 celeriac (celery roots), ends trimmed, chopped

3 cups (720 ml) Rosemary Beef Bone Broth (page 138) or store-bought beef broth

Preheat the oven to 450°F (230°C, or gas mark 8).

Place the beef roast in a large baking dish with a rack.

In a small bowl, whisk the oil, rosemary, garlic, thyme, salt, and pepper to taste. Rub the spice mixture onto the beef roast.

Arrange the vegetables in the baking dish around the roast. Pour the beef broth into the pan.

Bake the roast, uncovered, for 15 minutes. Reduce the heat to 325°F (160°C) and continue to bake the roast for about 1 hour more, or until the internal temperature reaches 125°F (52°C) for a rare roast, 130°F (55°C) for a medium-rare roast, or 135°F (58°C) for a medium roast. Let the roast rest for 10 minutes before slicing and serving.

Serve the roast with the vegetables and the broth poured over the top.

YIELD

8 SERVINGS

NUTRITIONAL ANALYSIS

PER SERVING (⅛ ROAST PLUS 1 CUP, WEIGHT VARIES, ROASTED VEGETABLES):

450 CALORIES

24G FAT

37G PROTEIN

24G CARBOHYDRATE

5G DIETARY FIBER

NOTE

Serve this dish with an appetizer salad or soup to make it the perfect pegan meal. I recommend light veggie-based options, like the Thai-Inspired Butternut Soup (page 61) or Summer Greek Salad (page 66). Keep it simple by adding a side of steamed greens, broccoli, or cauliflower.

CHAPTER 6

SIDE DISHES

The pegan diet is centered on a variety of low glycemic-load vegetables, so experimenting with a variety of vegetables and finding interesting ways to prepare them is key to beating boredom. Peruse your local farmers' markets and seek out less common vegetables to add to your meals.

CRISPY ROASTED BRUSSELS SPROUTS AND RADISHES

Roasting Brussels sprouts brings out a sweet, earthy quality that is absolutely addicting. This version adds radishes, which make a beautiful pairing. If you've never tried roasting radishes, the spicy flavor of the vegetable is replaced by a creamy sweetness. This dish pairs perfectly with simple meat dishes like Grilled Rosemary Pork Skewers (page 108) or Grass-Fed Roast Beef (page 118).

1 pound (454 g) Brussels sprouts, ends trimmed, halved

8 ounces (225 g) radishes, ends trimmed

2 tablespoons (30 ml) fresh lemon juice

1 tablespoon (15 ml) avocado oil

Sea salt and black pepper to taste

Preheat the oven to 450°F (230°C, or gas mark 8).

On a sheet pan, spread out the Brussels sprouts and radishes. Drizzle the vegetables with the lemon juice and oil. Season with salt and pepper to taste. Use your hands to toss the vegetables and coat them evenly in the seasonings.

Use your fingers to gently loosen the leaves around the edges from the Brussels sprouts. Allowing more air to circulate around the leaves makes the outer parts of the sprouts crunchier.

Roast the vegetables for 22 to 26 minutes until the Brussels sprout leaves are turning brown and crispy.

YIELD

6 SERVINGS

NUTRITIONAL ANALYSIS

PER SERVING:

145 CALORIES

6G FAT

4G PROTEIN

21G CARBOHYDRATE

7G DIETARY FIBER

NOTE

To maximize the crispy exterior of the sprouts, use your fingers to loosen the leaves on the outside of the sprouts before adding them to the sheet pan. I even rip some of the leaves off to let them brown and crisp more while baking.

ADD IT!

This simple recipe works well with a variety of veggies. Instead of radishes, add whatever you have on hand, such as parsnips, small cubed sweet potatoes, carrots, or cauliflower. The directions and seasonings remain the same.

CAULIFLOWER PARSNIP MASH

Mashed potatoes are an American classic. However, potatoes are very high on the glycemic index and are far from being the only vegetable that makes a delicious side dish. This lower-carb version uses a combination of cauliflower and parsnips, which results in a creamy, earthy, slightly sweet mash. You won't go back to regular potatoes after trying this delicious combo.

2 pounds (908 g) cauliflower, roughly chopped

1 pound (454 g) parsnips, ends trimmed, sliced

3 tablespoons (42 g) pastured butter

Sea salt and black pepper to taste

Place a steamer basket in a large pot and add at least 1 inch (2.5 cm) of water to the pot. Place the pot over medium-high heat. Place the cauliflower and parsnips in the steamer basket, cover, and steam for 15 to 20 minutes until soft. Drain the vegetables well and transfer them to a food processor.

Add the butter and salt and pepper to taste. Process until the vegetables are thick and smooth. Taste the mash and season with more salt and pepper, if necessary.

YIELD

6 SERVINGS

NUTRITIONAL ANALYSIS

PER SERVING:

145 CALORIES

6G FAT

4G PROTEIN

21G CARBOHYDRATE

7G DIETARY FIBER

NOTE

Parsnips look similar to carrots but are white and larger. They have a similar sweetness but are woodier in texture and are best served roasted or mashed. They are high in fiber as well as vitamins C, E, and K and folate. Although higher in carbs, they are a great way to switch up the veggies typically served in your kitchen.

ADD IT!

This basic cauliflower mash recipe can be made with a variety of vegetables. Cauliflower itself makes a watery mash, but adding a starchier vegetable, such as potato, parsnip, carrot, or celery root, makes a perfectly creamy, thick mash without adding any milk or liquid. Simply season the mash with butter, salt, and pepper.

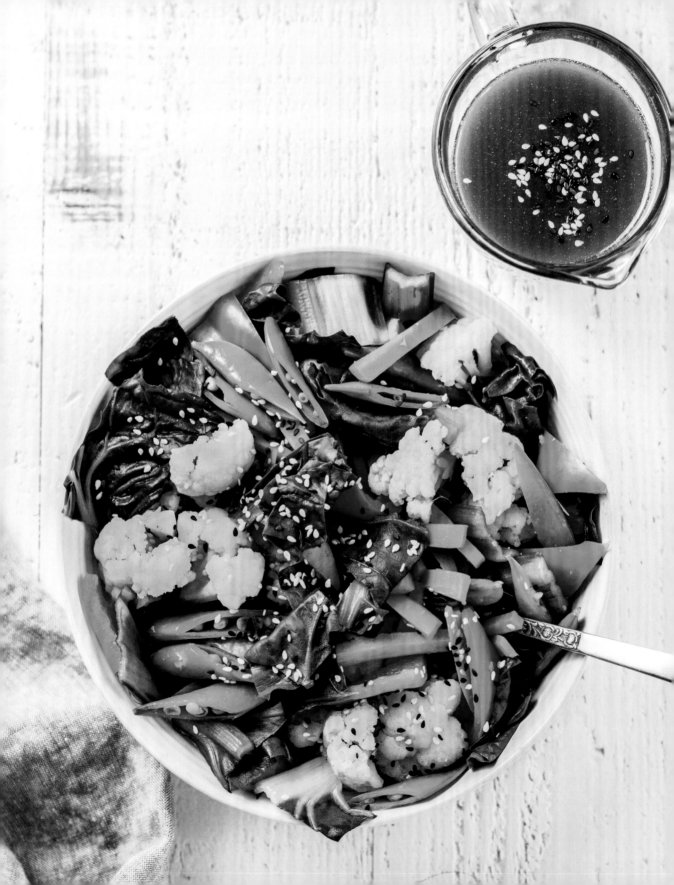

STEAMED ASIAN-STYLE VEGGIES WITH CLEAN TERIYAKI SAUCE

Steaming is one of the healthiest preparations for vegetables. When boiling vegetables, the nutrients leach into the water and are drained before eating. To jazz up steamed vegetables, this fun combination includes a tangy homemade teriyaki sauce. Serve these vegetables with poached salmon or chicken for a complete meal.

FOR STEAMED VEGETABLES:

3 cups (300 g) chopped cauliflower

2 cups (130 g) sugar snap peas, ends trimmed

1 carrot, sliced

1 red bell pepper, cored and sliced

6 cups (216 g) chopped rainbow chard with stems

FOR CLEAN TERIYAKI SAUCE:

6 tablespoons (90 ml) coconut aminos

2 tablespoons (30 ml) rice wine vinegar

2 tablespoons (30 ml) date syrup or (40 g) honey

1 tablespoon (15 ml) sesame oil

¼ teaspoon ground ginger

1 tablespoon (8 g) arrowroot powder

1 tablespoon (15 ml) water

YIELD

6 SERVINGS

NUTRITIONAL ANALYSIS

PER SERVING:

145 CALORIES

6G FAT

4G PROTEIN

21G CARBOHYDRATE

7G DIETARY FIBER

To make the steamed vegetables: Place a steamer basket in a large pot and add 1 inch (2.5 cm) of water to the pot. Place the pot over medium-high heat. Place the vegetables in the basket, cover, and steam for 5 to 7 minutes until crisp-tender.

To make the clean teriyaki sauce: In a small saucepan over medium heat, whisk the coconut aminos, vinegar, date syrup, oil, and ginger to combine. Cook for about 3 minutes until hot but not boiling.

In a small bowl, stir together the arrowroot powder and water until dissolved. Drizzle the slurry into the teriyaki mixture while whisking. Cook for about 1 minute to thicken, then remove from the heat.

Serve the steamed vegetables drizzled with the sauce.

NOTE

Coconut aminos is a popular substitute for soy sauce. Made from coconut tree sap, it is soy- and gluten-free and a healthy and safe substitution. Using a non-GMO organic tamari sauce is another option. To substitute tamari in this recipe, use ¼ cup (60 ml) tamari plus 2 tablespoons (30 ml) water in place of the coconut aminos.

ADD IT!

The teriyaki sauce in this recipe is perfect for drizzling on a wide range of veggies. It will jazz up plain steamed broccoli, or whatever veggies you have on hand to stir-fry or steam.

AUTUMN KALE SALAD

This nourishing salad celebrates the best produce of fall. It requires a bit of prep work, so I reserve salads like this for special occasions. Be sure to plan ahead and massage the kale in the dressing 4 to 8 hours before serving for the most flavorful results.

10 cups (670 g) chopped stemmed lacinato kale

½ cup (120 ml) Balsamic Dijon Vinaigrette (page 148)

1 delicata squash

1 tablespoon (15 ml) olive oil

Sea salt and black pepper to taste

1 golden beet

1 cup (180 g) pomegranate arils

½ cup (68 g) hazelnuts, toasted and roughly chopped

In a large salad bowl, combine the kale and vinaigrette. Use your hands to gently massage the dressing into the kale. This salad is best if this step is done 4 to 8 hours before serving. Cover the bowl and refrigerate until ready to serve.

Preheat the oven to 450°F (230°C, or gas mark 8). Line a large sheet pan with parchment or a silicone baking mat. Set aside.

Halve the squash lengthwise and scrape the seeds and pith from the center with a large spoon. Cut the squash halves into ½-inch (1 cm)-thick slices and place them on the prepared sheet pan. Drizzle or spray the squash with the oil and season with salt and pepper to taste.

Bake the squash for 15 to 20 minutes until browned on the bottom and soft throughout.

Bring a small pot full of water to a boil over high heat and add the beet. Turn the heat to medium and boil the beet for about 40 minutes, or until soft when pierced with a fork. Drain and let cool. Once cooled, the skin will peel off when pressed with your fingers. Halve the beet and cut it into thin half-rounds.

When ready to serve, transfer the kale to a large platter and top with the roasted squash and sliced beet. Top the salad with the pomegranate arils and hazelnuts.

YIELD

8 SERVINGS

NUTRITIONAL ANALYSIS

PER SERVING (1½ CUPS, WEIGHT VARIES):

195 CALORIES

12G FAT

6G PROTEIN

20G CARBOHYDRATE

3G DIETARY FIBER

ADD IT!

Add your favorite fall produce to this salad. Pears, apples, persimmons, and other squashes, like butternut, are delicious additions.

NOTE

When making special-occasion salads, I prep some of it ahead of time to streamline the process. I recommend making the vinaigrette, boiling the beet, toasting the hazelnuts, and peeling the pomegranate ahead of time.

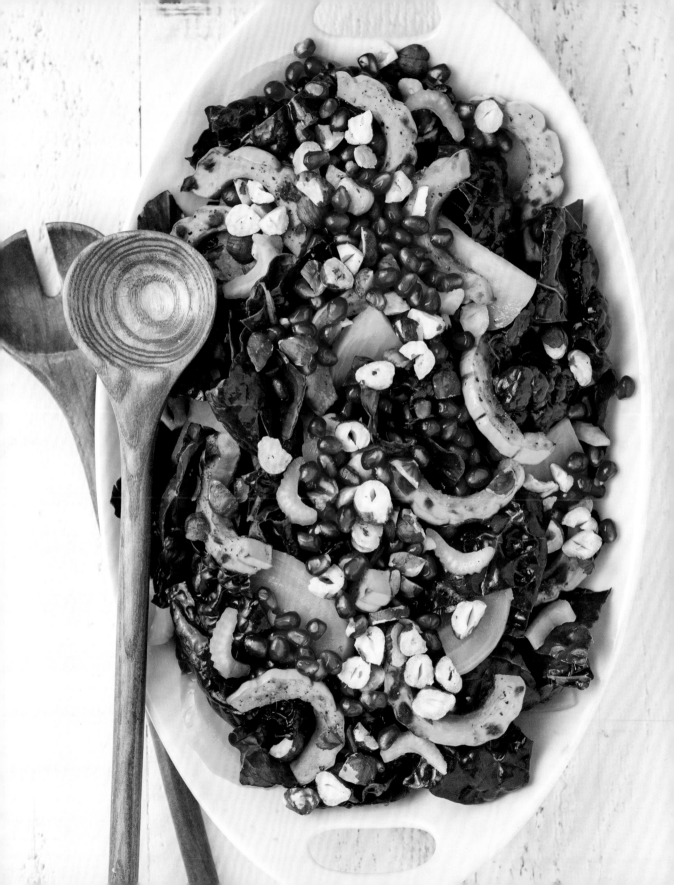

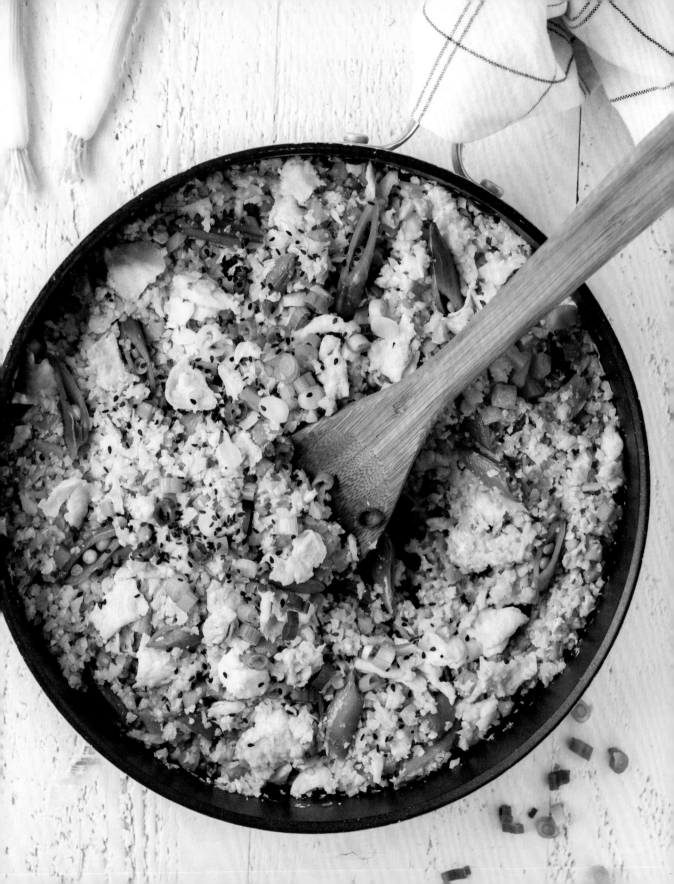

CAULIFLOWER FRIED RICE

Try this dish on a night you're craving take-out. Loaded with Asian flavors, this low-carb version is made with riced cauliflower. I make my own cauliflower rice because it tastes best fresh (and is the cheapest option), but if you're tight on time, keep frozen cauliflower rice on hand. Serve it as a light meal on its own, or add some protein to make a more filling meal.

1 pound (454 g) cauliflower florets

2 tablespoons (30 ml) sesame oil, divided

2 large eggs, beaten

1 carrot, diced

1 cup (65 g) sugar snap peas, ends trimmed, halved

6 tablespoons (90 ml) coconut aminos

1 teaspoon ground ginger

Pinch sea salt (optional)

Sliced scallions, for garnish (optional)

Rice the cauliflower by roughly chopping the florets and adding them to a food processor. Pulse until rice-size pieces form, without over-chopping it and making it too fine. Overprocessing the cauliflower will result in soggy cauliflower rice.

Heat a large skillet over high heat and add 1 tablespoon (15 ml) of the oil.

Add the beaten eggs and scramble them, slightly undercooking the eggs before removing them from the pan.

Return the skillet to the heat and add the remaining 1 tablespoon (15 ml) of oil, carrot, and peas. Sauté the vegetables for 3 to 4 minutes until softened.

Add the cauliflower rice to the skillet and stir-fry for about 5 minutes until heated through. Season the rice with the coconut aminos and ginger. Add a few pinches of salt to taste (if using).

Stir the egg back into the rice to combine. Serve garnished with scallions (if using).

YIELD

6 SERVINGS

NUTRITIONAL ANALYSIS

PER SERVING (1 CUP, WEIGHT VARIES):

108 CALORIES

6G FAT

4G PROTEIN

9G CARBOHYDRATE

2G DIETARY FIBER

ADD IT!

Add diced cooked leftover chicken, pork, or steak to make this a more complete meal, or double the amount of egg to add more protein.

CREAMY ASIAN-STYLE CUCUMBER NOODLES

A favorite side dish, these "noodles" can be a base to build a salad on. Especially refreshing on warm days, this fun use of cucumber is hydrating and full of sweet and sour flavor. Serve simply next to a prepared protein, like the Sesame-Ginger Grilled Chicken (page 99), or add slices of avocado and a hard-boiled egg for a quick and satiating lunch.

2 large English cucumbers

3 tablespoons (45 ml) unsweetened rice wine vinegar

2 tablespoons (30 g) tahini

2 tablespoons (30 ml) sesame oil

1 tablespoon (20 g) maple syrup

½ teaspoon sea salt

1 to 3 teaspoons (5 to 15 ml) paleo sriracha (optional)

2 tablespoons (16 g) toasted sesame seeds, or (12 g) toasted sliced almonds

Spiralize the cucumbers. If you do not have a spiralizer, use a vegetable peeler to make long fettuccini-style noodles, peeling lengthwise down the cucumber. Add the noodles to a large salad bowl.

In a lidded jar, combine the vinegar, tahini, oil, maple syrup, salt, and sriracha (if using). Cover the jar and shake vigorously until a smooth and creamy dressing forms.

Pour the dressing over the cucumber noodles and toss to coat and combine. Top with the toasted sesame seeds to serve.

YIELD

4 SERVINGS

NUTRITIONAL ANALYSIS

PER SERVING (½ CUCUMBER AND 2 TABLESPOONS, OR 30 ML, DRESSING):

154 CALORIES

13G FAT

3G PROTEIN

8G CARBOHYDRATE

2G DIETARY FIBER

ADD IT!

These noodles are a great base to build a quick meal on. Some of my favorite combos are leftover chicken, orange slices, and toasted almonds, or salmon, avocado, and sliced red bell pepper. Get creative and build your perfect noodle bowl.

ROASTED RAINBOW CARROTS

Choosing less common produce, like rainbow-hued carrots, is a great way to reap additional nutritional benefits from your diet. Each color contains different antioxidants, meaning more variety on your plate. This easy preparation results in sweet, tender carrots—a perfect side dish for any night of the week.

1½ pounds (681 g) rainbow carrots, tops trimmed

1 tablespoon (15 ml) avocado oil

½ teaspoon sea salt

1 tablespoon (3 g) fresh thyme leaves, or ½ teaspoon dried thyme

Black pepper to taste

Preheat the oven to 425°F (220°C, or gas mark 7).

Arrange the carrots on a large sheet pan. Drizzle with the oil and season with the salt, thyme, and pepper to taste.

Roast the carrots for 25 minutes until soft.

YIELD

6 SERVINGS

NUTRITIONAL ANALYSIS

PER SERVING (ABOUT 2 CARROTS):

67 CALORIES

3G FAT

1G PROTEIN

11G CARBOHYDRATE

3G DIETARY FIBER

NOTE

Rainbow carrots are often sold with their green tops attached. The greens are edible, so save them. I often throw them into my Waste-Not Vegetable Broth (page 139), but you can also throw them into a pesto or add to grain salads similar to using parsley. The best way to make a pegan diet more economical is to use all the edible parts of your food.

MEDITERRANEAN SAUTÉED ARTICHOKE HEARTS

Artichoke hearts are an often-forgotten vegetable, but there's good reason to bring them back to your plate. They are high in fiber and listed as the seventh highest food in antioxidants. This easy dish is made with canned or jarred artichoke hearts, meaning you can enjoy them more often. Serve this dish hot, or chill it and serve cold. It's delicious either way.

2 tablespoons (30 ml) olive oil

5 garlic cloves, minced

2 (14-ounce, or 395 g) cans artichoke hearts in water, drained and quartered

1 cup (100 g) quartered pitted olives

¼ cup (30 g) chopped oil-packed sun-dried tomatoes

1 tablespoon (15 ml) fresh lemon juice

1 tablespoon (15 ml) balsamic vinegar

¼ cup (34 g) pine nuts

¼ cup (10 g) chopped fresh basil

¼ cup (16 g) chopped fresh Italian parsley

Heat a large skillet over medium heat and add the oil and garlic. Sauté the garlic for a few minutes until it begins to brown. Lower the heat to medium-low.

Add the artichoke hearts, olives, and sun-dried tomatoes. Gently stir-fry for about 5 minutes until the vegetables are heated through. Transfer the vegetables to a serving dish and drizzle with the lemon juice and vinegar. Garnish with the pine nuts, basil, and Italian parsley.

Refrigerate leftovers in an airtight container for up to 5 days.

YIELD

8 SERVINGS

NUTRITIONAL ANALYSIS

PER SERVING (½ CUP, ABOUT 130 G):

108 CALORIES

9G FAT

2G PROTEIN

6G CARBOHYDRATE

2G DIETARY FIBER

NOTE

If it's possible, find artichoke hearts packed in a glass jar. Otherwise, look for cans with a non-BPA liner. This recipe uses artichoke hearts in water. If you have marinated artichoke hearts on hand, skip the lemon juice and vinegar in the recipe.

NOTE

This dish is versatile. Enjoy it as a vegetable side dish, as a topper for chicken or fish, or even add it to wraps and salads. I love having a container of this in the refrigerator to add flavor and fiber to simple meals.

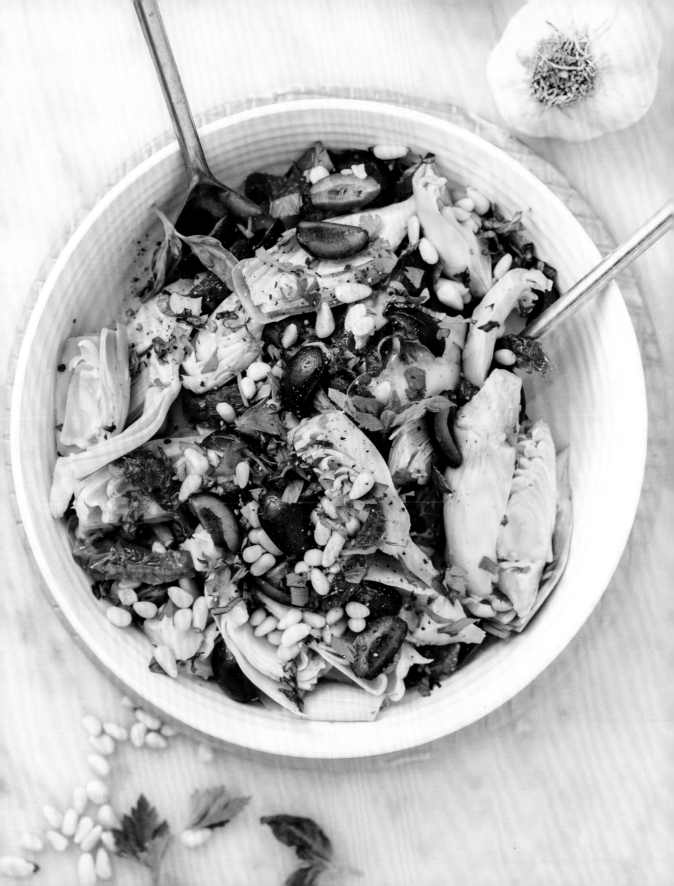

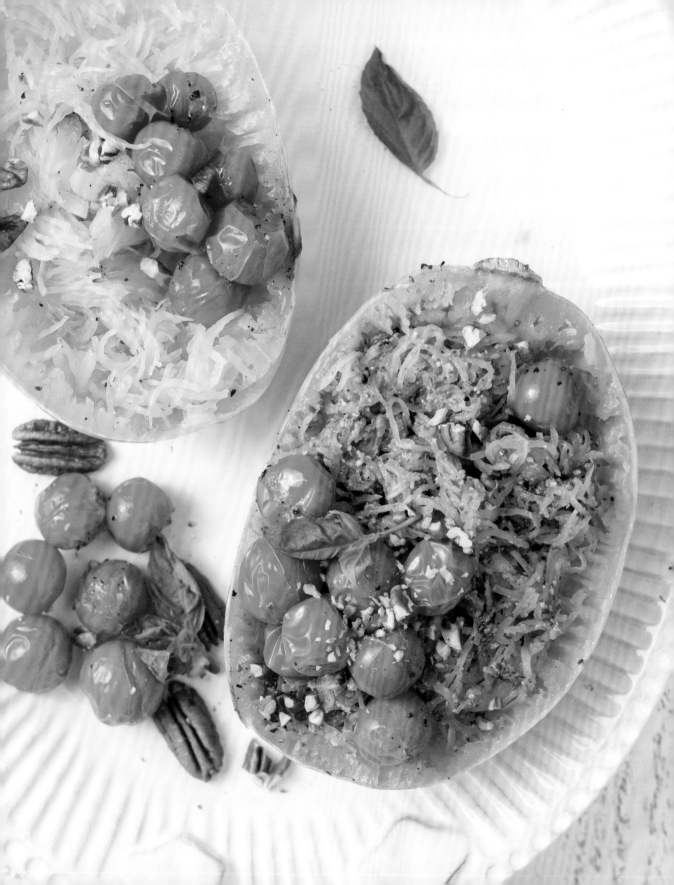

PESTO SPAGHETTI SQUASH WITH BLISTERED TOMATOES

Spaghetti squash is a delicious vegetable that makes a great stand-in for high glycemic, low-nutrient pastas. You can dress it up any way you would a pasta dish. This fun version uses roasted spaghetti squash tossed in pesto and topped with blistered cherry tomatoes. Add roasted chicken, fish, or a fried egg to complete the meal.

1 (about 4-pound, or 1.8 kg) spaghetti squash

2 tablespoons (30 ml) avocado oil, divided

Sea salt and black pepper to taste

2 cups (298 g) cherry tomatoes

½ cup (120 g) Pecan Arugula Pesto (page 145), plus more as needed

Preheat the oven to 400°F (200°C, or gas mark 6).

Halve the spaghetti squash and use a large spoon to dig out the seeds. Rub the cut side of the squash with 1 tablespoon (15 ml) of the oil and lightly season with salt and pepper to taste. Place the squash halves, cut-side down, on a sheet pan.

Bake the squash for 40 minutes to 1 hour, depending on the size of the squash. The squash is ready when the strands easily pull away from the skin but don't easily fall apart. Remove the squash from the sheet pan.

Place the tomatoes on the sheet pan and toss with the remaining 1 tablespoon (15 ml) of oil. Season with salt and pepper, if desired.

Bake the tomatoes for 10 minutes until the skins burst.

Use a fork to gently scoop the squash strands from the skins and place them in a large bowl. Add the pesto and toss to coat. If your spaghetti squash is larger than 4 pounds, use more pesto to taste.

Serve the pesto spaghetti squash topped with the blistered tomatoes.

YIELD

7 SERVINGS

NUTRITIONAL ANALYSIS

PER SERVING (1 CUP, WEIGHT VARIES):

169 CALORIES

12G FAT

2G PROTEIN

16G CARBOHYDRATE

3G DIETARY FIBER

NOTE

Use your favorite store-bought pesto to save time. The Pecan Arugula Pesto (page 145) recommended in this recipe is dairy-free and uses heart-healthy cashews rather than cheese. If seeking a quality store-bought option, look for a vegan version that uses olive oil rather than refined vegetable oils.

SAUTÉED BEET GREENS

Don't throw away the greens on top of your beets. Beet greens are just as delicious as the root vegetables themselves and one of the healthiest foods we can eat. They burst with vitamin K, calcium, copper, and iron. I typically prepare these the day I buy beets so they are fresh, knowing the beets themselves will be fine for weeks in the refrigerator.

1 bunch (270 g) beet greens

2 tablespoons (28 g) pastured butter

1 shallot, minced

¼ teaspoon sea salt

3 tablespoons (45 ml) dry white wine

1 tablespoon (20 g) maple syrup (optional)

¼ cup (34 g) pine nuts, toasted

1 tablespoon (8 g) sesame seeds, toasted

Thoroughly wash and roughly chop the beet greens and set aside.

Heat a large skillet over medium heat and add the butter, shallot, and salt. Sauté for about 7 minutes until the shallot is softened and beginning to brown.

Stir in the white wine and maple syrup (if using). Turn the heat to medium-low and simmer for about 10 minutes until most of the liquid is reduced.

Add the beet greens and stir to coat in the shallot reduction. Cover the skillet and steam the greens for 3 to 5 minutes until softened.

Serve the greens garnished with the pine nuts and sesame seeds.

YIELD

4 SERVINGS

NUTRITIONAL ANALYSIS

PER SERVING (½ CUP, OR 70 G, COOKED GREENS):

287 CALORIES

13G FAT

25G PROTEIN

17G CARBOHYDRATE

3G DIETARY FIBER

NOTE

Beet greens are versatile. Add chopped greens to the Steamed Asian-Style Veggies with Clean Teriyaki Sauce (page 123) or freeze and add to smoothies and soups. If nothing else, save them to make Waste-Not Vegetable Broth (page 139) or Rosemary Beef Bone Broth (page 138).

CHAPTER 7

◆ ◆ ◆

GRAVY, BROTHS, DIPS, SAUCES, AND DRESSINGS

Most store-bought condiments are filled with sugar, additives, and preservatives, in addition to being made with low-quality or refined oils. Making your own is easy to do and you can be choosy with the ingredients.

APPLE-SAGE TURKEY GRAVY

Gravy has gotten a bad rap for the wrong reasons. The drippings from pastured poultry are nutritious and add a ton of flavor to meats and veggies. This easy gravy recipe uses egg yolks rather than starch to thicken it. Use this recipe with turkey or chicken drippings.

1 cup (240 ml) turkey drippings

1 apple, cored and chopped, or ½ cup (120 ml) unfiltered apple juice

2 large egg yolks

1 tablespoon (3 g) finely chopped fresh sage

½ teaspoon Dijon mustard

Sea salt and black pepper to taste

Add the drippings to a small saucepan.

In a blender or food processor, process the apple until it is broken up. Transfer the pulp to a piece of cheesecloth or a nut milk bag and squeeze the juice into a bowl. You can substitute store-bought unfiltered apple juice and omit this step. Set the apple juice aside.

In a small bowl, combine ¼ cup (60 ml) of the drippings from the pan, once they are somewhat cool (warm is okay) and the egg yolks. Whisk to blend. Pour the mixture into the pan with the turkey drippings. Turn the heat to medium and whisk while gently heating.

Whisk in the apple juice and cook, whisking, for 2 to 3 minutes more. Remove from the heat before the gravy begins to boil.

Whisk in the sage and Dijon. Taste and season with salt and pepper to taste.

Refrigerate leftovers in an airtight container for up to 1 week.

YIELD

6 SERVINGS

NUTRITIONAL ANALYSIS

PER SERVING (¼ CUP, OR 60 ML):

341 CALORIES

34G FAT

1G PROTEIN

3G CARBOHYDRATE

0G DIETARY FIBER

NOTE

This method works with fatty drippings from roasted chicken or turkey but does not work with chicken or turkey stock, which is mostly water. The fat from the egg yolks easily blends with high-fat drippings but will not blend into a watery base.

ANTI-INFLAMMATORY CHICKEN BONE BROTH

Bone broth has recently gained popularity for good reason. When we throw away a chicken carcass, we lose valuable nutrients. The marrow, collagen, and connective tissues in chicken bones are rich in glycine, which is known to regulate blood sugar levels, improve muscle repair and growth, boost mood, and reduce stress. This flavorful version uses turmeric and ginger, both known for their anti-inflammatory properties, to give this broth double the healing power. Drink this broth, or use it as a base for soups.

1 whole chicken carcass, meat removed and saved for another use

1 pound (454 g) chicken wings

8 cups (1.9 L) water, or more as needed

¾ cup (75 g) roughly chopped peeled fresh ginger

2 shallots, roughly chopped

1 tablespoon (15 ml) rice wine vinegar

1½ teaspoons ground turmeric

Sea salt to taste

In a slow cooker, combine the carcass, wings, water, ginger, shallots, vinegar, and turmeric. Cover the cooker and set it to High heat until a low simmer is reached. Reduce the heat to Low and cook for 16 to 24 hours.

If necessary, replace evaporated water about three-fourths of the way through the cooking time.

Strain the broth through a fine-mesh sieve set over a heatproof bowl. Taste and season the broth with salt to taste. Let cool, then transfer to glass jars.

Refrigerate the broth in tightly sealed glass jars for 4 to 5 days, or freeze for up to 3 months.

YIELD

6 SERVINGS

NUTRITIONAL ANALYSIS

PER SERVING (1 CUP, OR 240 ML):

41 CALORIES

0.5G FAT

10G PROTEIN

0.5G CARBOHYDRATE

0G DIETARY FIBER

NOTE

Freeze individual servings of this broth and keep them on hand for when someone in the family gets sick. If the flavor and texture are difficult to get used to, try mixing the bone broth with chicken stock in a 50:50 ratio and lessen the amount of stock over time.

ADD IT!

Omit the ginger, turmeric, and shallots and replace them with onion, garlic, celery, and rosemary sprigs for a different flavor, still full of healing properties. Whatever you choose, use a lot of flavoring. Bone broth doesn't taste like traditional chicken stock, so adding lots of flavor helps it be more palatable.

ROSEMARY BEEF BONE BROTH

Like chicken bone broth (see Anti-Inflammatory Chicken Bone Broth, page 137), beef bone broth is another healing drink, full of collagen and omega-3 fatty acids. Western diets, often, do not benefit from the connective tissues and bone marrow of beef cuts, which are arguably more nutritious than muscle meat. Bone broth is an easy way to extract nutrients and benefit from the entire animal.

2 pounds (908 g) grass-fed beef bones

Avocado oil

12 cups (2.9 L) water

2 tablespoons (30 ml) apple cider vinegar

1 tablespoon (15 g) sea salt

1 head garlic, roughly chopped

1 onion, quartered

2 celery stalks

5 rosemary sprigs

Preheat the oven to 400°F (200°C, or gas mark 6).

Place the beef bones on a large sheet pan and lightly spray or brush with oil.

Roast the bones for 15 minutes, flip them, and roast for 15 minutes more until the bones have taken on a toasted color. Transfer the bones to a slow cooker and add the water, vinegar, salt, garlic, vegetables, and rosemary.

Cover the cooker and cook on Low heat for 12 to 24 hours.

Strain the broth through a fine-mesh sieve set over a heatproof bowl. Let cool, then transfer to glass jars.

Refrigerate the broth in tightly sealed glass jars for 4 to 5 days, or freeze for up to 3 months.

YIELD

20 SERVINGS

NUTRITIONAL ANALYSIS

PER SERVING (1 CUP, OR 240 ML):

70 CALORIES

4G FAT

6G PROTEIN

0.5G CARBOHYDRATE

0G DIETARY FIBER

NOTE

The rich and fatty texture of bone broth can be difficult to adjust to if you imagine it tasting similar to canned beef broth. To begin drinking bone broth, mix it with beef or vegetable stock in a 50:50 ratio and season it with salt and pepper.

ADD IT!

Save vegetable trimmings in a container in the freezer and pull them out to flavor bone broth. Instead of using the onion, garlic, and celery, substitute whatever trimmings you've saved. Be sure to add ample seasonings.

WASTE-NOT VEGETABLE BROTH

If buying organic vegetables, save the trimmings and unused parts and turn them into a nutrient-rich soup base. I keep a large storage container in my freezer and fill it with the stems and peels of my vegetables throughout the week. When it's full, the trimmings are simmered to make a flavorful, healthy broth. This broth is not only more flavorful than store-bought versions, but it's also a great way to stretch your grocery budget and reduce food waste.

2 pounds (908 g) vegetable trimmings

1 onion, skin on, quartered

1 head garlic, skin on, roughly chopped

4 rosemary sprigs

4 thyme sprigs

10 cups (2.4 L) water

Sea salt and black pepper to taste

In a slow cooker, combine the trimmings, onion, garlic, rosemary, thyme, and water. Cover the cooker and set it to High heat until a low simmer is reached. Reduce the heat to Low and cook for 4 to 6 hours.

If necessary, replace the evaporated water about three-fourths of the way through the cooking time.

Strain the broth through a fine-mesh sieve set over a heatproof bowl. Taste and season the broth with salt and pepper to taste. Let cool, then transfer to glass jars.

Refrigerate the broth in tightly sealed glass jars for 4 to 5 days, or freeze for up to 3 months.

YIELD

10 SERVINGS

NUTRITIONAL ANALYSIS

PER SERVING (1 CUP, OR 240 ML):

13 CALORIES

0G FAT

0.5 G PROTEIN

2G CARBOHYDRATE

0G DIETARY FIBER

NOTE

Use only organic vegetables for a homemade broth because the discarded parts of vegetables (such as the peels) are typically those most affected by pesticides. Thoroughly wash the vegetables before preparing them and add all unused parts of the vegetables, such as leaves, stems, seeds, and peels to your storage container in the freezer. I like to add fresh onion, garlic, thyme, and rosemary to punch up the flavor of the broth, but use any herbs you have on hand.

ROASTED CARROT HUMMUS

Carrots are roasted to bring out their natural sweetness, then puréed with all the traditional hummus ingredients. This dip is a great replacement for those looking to cut out or reduce legumes in their diet. Garnish this hummus with crunchy toasted pumpkin seeds or pomegranate arils for added texture.

2 pounds (908 g) carrots, cut into sticks

1 tablespoon (15 ml) avocado oil

6 tablespoons (90 g) tahini

3 tablespoons (45 g) fresh lemon juice

2 tablespoons (30 g) olive oil

½ teaspoon sea salt

1 garlic clove, peeled

4 cinnamon sticks

Preheat the oven to 400°F (200°C, or gas mark 6). Line a sheet pan with parchment paper or a silicone baking mat.

Arrange the carrots in a single layer on the prepared sheet pan. Drizzle the carrots with the avocado oil and toss to coat.

Bake the carrots for 30 to 35 minutes until very soft. Transfer the carrots to a food processor.

Add the tahini, lemon juice, olive oil, and salt to the processor. Process for 3 to 4 minutes, stopping to scrape down the sides every minute or so, until the mixture is light and the carrots are fully processed.

Grate the garlic into the hummus and pulse it in. Transfer the warm hummus to an airtight storage container and press the cinnamon sticks into the mixture. Chill for a couple of hours, up to overnight. Remove the cinnamon sticks and stir well before serving.

Refrigerate leftovers in an airtight container for up to 1 week.

YIELD

6 SERVINGS

NUTRITIONAL ANALYSIS

PER SERVING (½ CUP, OR 112 G):

108 CALORIES

8G FAT

2G PROTEIN

9G CARBOHYDRATE

2G DIETARY FIBER

NOTE

This delicious legume-free twist on hummus is not lacking in flavor. Use this however you'd use a traditional hummus—as a dip, a spread, or a salad topper.

BABA GHANOUSH

This earthy, flavorful dip is similar to hummus but made with roasted eggplant rather than chickpeas. The Mediterranean classic is rich in fiber, vitamin E, and zinc. It's a perfect salad topper, spread, or veggie dip. Keep this on hand for healthy snacking.

2 pounds (908 g) eggplant

Avocado oil

⅓ cup (90 g) tahini

¼ cup (60 ml) olive oil

2 tablespoons (30 ml) fresh lemon juice, plus more for seasoning

¾ teaspoon sea salt, plus more for seasoning

¼ teaspoon ground cumin

2 garlic cloves, peeled

Chopped fresh Italian parsley, for garnish

Preheat the oven to 450°F (230°C, or gas mark 8). Line a sheet pan with parchment paper.

Halve the eggplant lengthwise and spray or brush it with avocado oil. Place the eggplant, cut-side down, on the prepared sheet pan.

Bake the eggplant for 30 to 35 minutes until the flesh is softened and creamy. Scoop out the flesh to remove it from the skin and transfer it to a food processor.

Add the tahini, olive oil, lemon juice, salt, and cumin. Process the mixture until it's very smooth and lightens in color.

Grate the garlic into the dip, tasting and adjusting the salt and lemon juice, if necessary. Process to mix in the garlic and seasonings fully. Chill before serving. Serve garnished with parsley.

Refrigerate leftovers in an airtight container for up to 1 week.

YIELD

8 SERVINGS

NUTRITIONAL ANALYSIS

PER SERVING (¼ CUP, OR 56 G):

150 CALORIES

12G FAT

3G PROTEIN

9G CARBOHYDRATE

4G DIETARY FIBER

NOTE

Serve this dip with cut vegetables, such as carrots, bell peppers, cucumber, or cauliflower. It is also delicious used as a spread for the Garlic and Rosemary Almond Meal Flaxseed Crackers (page 40).

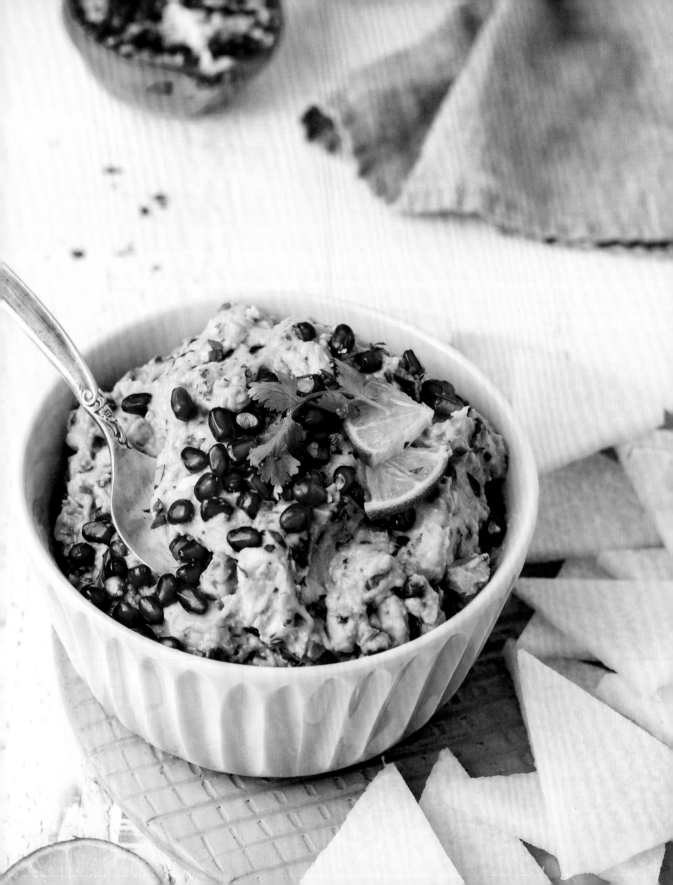

POMEGRANATE GUACAMOLE

A festive, bright guacamole recipe with pops of sweetness from the pomegranate arils, this healthy party appetizer is a great dip, spread, or topping for grilled meats or salads. Pomegranates are loaded with important nutrients such as fiber, vitamins C and K, folate, and potassium, so find creative uses for this fruit.

3 ripe avocados

1½ cups (270 g) pomegranate arils

**1 jalapeño pepper, minced,
   or to taste**

¼ cup (4 g) chopped fresh cilantro

**¼ cup (60 ml) fresh lime juice,
   plus more for storing leftovers**

**3 tablespoons (45 ml) fresh
   orange juice**

½ teaspoon salt, or to taste

⅛ teaspoon ground cumin

Halve the avocados and scoop the flesh into a medium-size bowl. Use a fork to mash the avocados, leaving some chunks for added texture, if desired.

Stir in the pomegranate arils, jalapeño, cilantro, lime juice, orange juice, salt, and cumin, mixing well.

Taste and season with salt, if needed, or adjust the heat with more jalapeño, if desired. Serve immediately.

Sprinkle lime juice over any leftovers and refrigerate in an airtight container, with a piece of plastic pressed into the top of the guacamole to create a barrier between the avocado and the air, for 1 to 2 days.

YIELD

7 SERVINGS

NUTRITIONAL ANALYSIS

PER SERVING (½ CUP, OR 112 G):

171 CALORIES

13G FAT

2G PROTEIN

15G CARBOHYDRATE

7G DIETARY FIBER

NOTE

Although pomegranate is the star of this guacamole, this fruit is not available year-round. If you find yourself craving some fruity guacamole in spring or summer, try chopped strawberries or peaches in place of the pomegranate.

CHIMICHURRI

One of my favorite condiments, chimichurri is a South American pesto. Although many modern versions use cilantro, the traditional version has a base of parsley. Using chimichurri on your steak instead of steak sauce is a great way to freshen up a plate while also adding nutrients.

1 cup (60 g) fresh Italian parsley

1 tablespoon (2 g) fresh thyme leaves

2 tablespoons (30 ml) olive oil

2 tablespoons (30 ml) red wine vinegar

1 tablespoon (15 ml) fresh lemon juice

1 garlic clove, minced

½ teaspoon sea salt

¼ teaspoon paprika

¼ teaspoon red pepper flakes

On a cutting board, use a large knife to chop the parsley and thyme very finely. Transfer the herbs to a small bowl. Stir in the remaining ingredients, mixing well.

Refrigerate leftovers in an airtight container for 1 to 3 days.

YIELD

8 SERVINGS

NUTRITIONAL ANALYSIS

PER SERVING (2 TABLESPOONS, OR 30 G):

109 CALORIES

11G FAT

1G PROTEIN

2G CARBOHYDRATE

1G DIETARY FIBER

NOTE

Chimichurri is most commonly served with steak, but it is a delicious complement to seafood such as salmon and shrimp. The bright flavors are also perfectly paired with roasted potatoes and sweet vegetables, like squash and carrots.

PECAN ARUGULA PESTO

A delicious and nutritious twist on the staple Italian condiment, this pesto features peppery arugula and sweet pecans. This version is kept dairy-free using cashews in place of the traditional Parmesan cheese. Use this as an accompaniment to vegetables and meats, or try it as a salad topper.

2 cups (40 g) arugula

2 cups (70 g) fresh basil leaves

¼ cup (28 g) toasted pecans

¼ cup (35 g) raw cashews

¼ cup (60 ml) olive oil

2½ tablespoons (38 ml) fresh lemon juice

2 tablespoons (30 ml) water, plus more as needed

1 garlic clove, peeled

¼ teaspoon sea salt, or to taste

Black pepper to taste

In a food processor, combine the arugula and basil. Process to chop the greens.

Add the pecans and cashews and pulse to break up the nuts.

With the processor running, drizzle in the oil, lemon juice, and water, creating a green paste. Thin with an additional tablespoon or two (15 to 30 ml) of water, if desired.

Grate the garlic into the pesto. Add salt and pepper to taste and pulse to mix.

Refrigerate the pesto in an airtight container for up to 1 week, or freeze for up to 3 months.

YIELD

8 SERVINGS

NUTRITIONAL ANALYSIS

PER SERVING (2 TABLESPOONS, OR 30 G):

109 CALORIES

11G FAT

1G PROTEIN

2G CARBOHYDRATE

1G DIETARY FIBER

NOTE

Arugula is a peppery green that is both extremely nutritious and delicious. It's a cruciferous vegetable in the same family as broccoli and cauliflower and provides many of the same nutritional benefits.

MUSHROOM CREAM SAUCE

This super creamy mushroom- and garlic-studded sauce is completely dairy-free. Puréed cashews and cauliflower make a thick and flavorful base, perfect for enhancing with your favorite add-ins. It's delicious for topping chicken or steak or adding to a side of steamed wild rice or quinoa.

1 cup (140 g) raw cashews

2 cups (200 g) chopped cauliflower

¾ to 1 cup (180 to 240 ml) water

1 tablespoon (14 g) pastured butter

2 garlic cloves, minced

1 pound (454 g) mushrooms, sliced

2 teaspoons fresh thyme leaves

1 teaspoon sea salt

Black pepper to taste

Soak the cashews in water and cover overnight.

Place a steamer basket in a large pot and add 1 inch (2.5 cm) of water to the pot. Place the pot over medium-high heat. Place the cauliflower in the basket, cover, and steam for about 15 minutes until the cauliflower breaks apart with a fork. Drain and transfer the cauliflower to a blender.

Drain and rinse the cashews and add them to the blender with ¾ cup (180 ml) of water. Process for 3 to 4 minutes until a very smooth sauce forms. If needed, add the remaining ¼ cup (60 ml) of water, a little at a time, if the sauce is too thick.

Heat a large skillet over medium heat and add the butter and garlic. Sauté the garlic for about 5 minutes, then add the mushrooms, cashew-cauliflower mixture, thyme, salt, and pepper to taste. Cook for about 10 minutes until the mushrooms are soft, stirring occasionally.

Refrigerate leftovers in an airtight container for up to 3 days. Do not freeze. To reheat, thin with a little water and warm over medium-low heat, stirring frequently.

NOTE

Cutting dairy from your diet does not mean going without creamy sauces. Cashews and cauliflower both make great stand-ins for dairy and add fiber and potassium to dishes. This versatile sauce can be made for a variety of uses or even transformed into a cream of mushroom soup by thinning it with vegetable broth.

YIELD

6 SERVINGS

NUTRITIONAL ANALYSIS

PER SERVING (½ CUP, OR 120 ML):

163 CALORIES

12G FAT

7G PROTEIN

11G CARBOHYDRATE

2G DIETARY FIBER

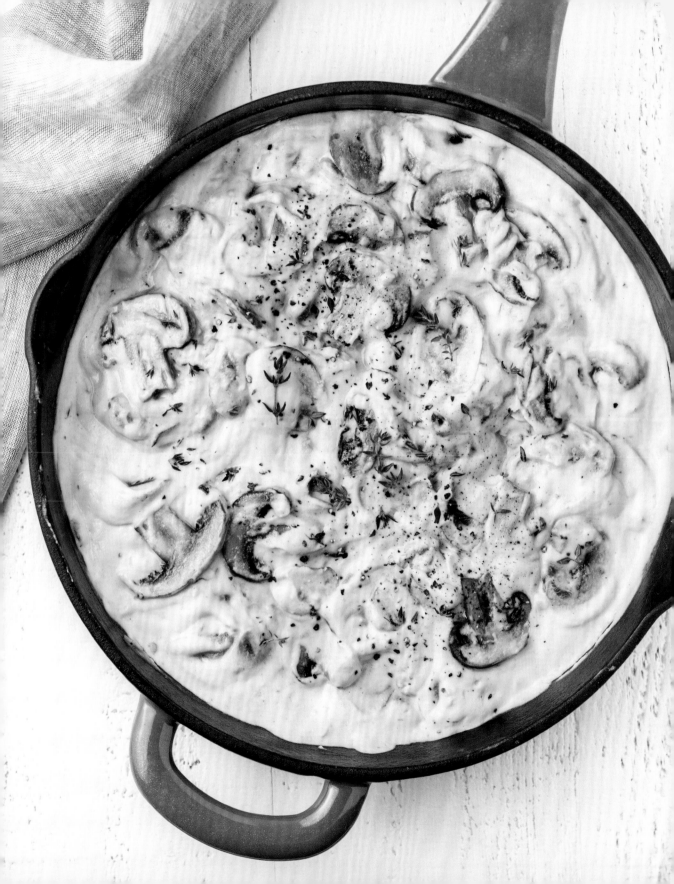

EASY LEMON VINAIGRETTE

I rely on this dressing more than any other condiment. It adds a bright splash of citrus and works as a salad dressing as well as a meat marinade. I also use it to pull together grain and vegetable salads, like the Moroccan-Style Chickpea Salad (page 75). It will become a staple in your refrigerator, like mine. True simplicity at its best.

½ cup (120 ml) fresh lemon juice

½ cup (120 ml) olive oil

3 tablespoons (45 ml) white wine vinegar

1 teaspoon (4 g) Dijon mustard

Sea salt and black pepper to taste

In a blender or jar, combine all the dressing ingredients and process, or cover the jar and shake, until the dressing is fully mixed.

Refrigerate in an airtight container for up to 1 month.

YIELD

9 SERVINGS

NUTRITIONAL ANALYSIS

PER SERVING
(2 TABLESPOONS,
OR 30 ML):

110 CALORIES

12G FAT

1G PROTEIN

1G CARBOHYDRATE

1G DIETARY FIBER

NOTE

If you prefer a sweeter dressing, add 1 to 2 tablespoons (20 to 40 g) of maple syrup. I find that using this dressing on salads with sweet toppings, like fruit, carrots, or beets, is enough.

BALSAMIC DIJON VINAIGRETTE

This is a classic salad dressing that takes minutes to put together and is a great multipurpose condiment. Having flavorful dressings already made helps me choose salads over convenience foods on busy days. The sweet flavor of balsamic pairs well with a variety of salad toppings—from meats to fruit and olives.

½ cup (120 ml) balsamic vinegar

½ cup (120 ml) olive oil

1 tablespoon (2 g) fresh thyme leaves, or 1 teaspoon dried thyme

1 teaspoon Dijon mustard

Sea salt and black pepper to taste

In a blender, combine all the dressing ingredients and process until thick and creamy. The color will change to a creamy brown.

Refrigerate in an airtight container for up to 1 month.

YIELD

8 SERVINGS

NUTRITIONAL ANALYSIS

PER SERVING
(2 TABLESPOONS,
OR 30 ML):

134 CALORIES

14G FAT

1G PROTEIN

3G CARBOHYDRATE

0G DIETARY FIBER

NOTE

Save time by making this dressing in a jar and shaking to combine. I prefer to process it in a blender to emulsify the dressing and get a creamy texture, but either method works.

SPICY AVOCADO-CILANTRO DRESSING

Perfect for taco salads, dipping veggies, or even adding dollops of flavor to chicken, pork or steak dishes, this avocado dressing will have you hooked. I love tossing crunchy romaine lettuce with this, then topping it with chicken, olives, and chopped tomatoes for a quick, healthy, and completely satisfying meal.

½ avocado, pitted, flesh scooped from the skin

½ cup (120 ml) water

3 tablespoons (45 ml) fresh lime juice

1 tablespoon (16 g) cashew butter

½ teaspoon sea salt

¼ teaspoon ground cumin

⅓ cup (5 g) chopped fresh cilantro

1 to 2 tablespoons (9 to 18 g) chopped jalapeño pepper, plus more for seasoning

In a blender, combine the avocado, water, lime juice, cashew butter, salt, and cumin. Process until smooth.

Add the cilantro and jalapeño and pulse to incorporate. Taste and adjust the heat with more jalapeño, if desired.

Refrigerate in an airtight container for up to 4 days.

YIELD

8 SERVINGS

NUTRITIONAL ANALYSIS

PER SERVING (2 TABLESPOONS, OR 30 ML):

35 CALORIES

3G FAT

1G PROTEIN

2G CARBOHYDRATE

1G DIETARY FIBER

NOTE

Think of this as a thinned-out guacamole, perfect for drizzling anywhere you'd usually use the popular Mexican dip. My family loves this on Kale Taco Salad (page 111).

ADD IT!

Add a sweet and spicy twist to this dressing using ½ cup (120 ml) of fresh orange juice in place of the water.

THAI-INSPIRED ALMOND SALAD DRESSING

Warning: This dressing will cause salad cravings. An irresistible blend of almond butter and Asian flavors is enough to tempt even the most veggie-weary people. Toss simple romaine lettuce with this dressing, or use it to dip chicken satay-style, or create your own Thai-style chicken lettuce wraps with this fun-to-drizzle dressing.

¼ cup (65 g) almond butter

¼ cup (60 ml) full-fat coconut milk

¼ cup (60 ml) unsweetened rice wine vinegar

3 tablespoons (45 ml) coconut aminos

1 tablespoon (15 ml) sesame oil

1 tablespoon (15 ml) fresh lime juice

1 to 2 teaspoons paleo sriracha, plus more for seasoning

¼ to ½ teaspoon sea salt, plus more for seasoning

In a blender, combine all the dressing ingredients and process until a light and creamy dressing forms. Taste and add more sriracha and salt, as desired.

Refrigerate in an airtight container for up to 1 week.

YIELD

8 SERVINGS

NUTRITIONAL ANALYSIS

PER SERVING (2 TABLESPOONS, OR 30 ML):

68 CALORIES

6G FAT

1G PROTEIN

2G CARBOHYDRATE

1G DIETARY FIBER

NOTE

Coconut aminos is a soy sauce substitute that is both soy- and gluten-free. It is made from coconut tree sap, and combined with salt, has a lightly sweet flavor similar to the traditional condiment.

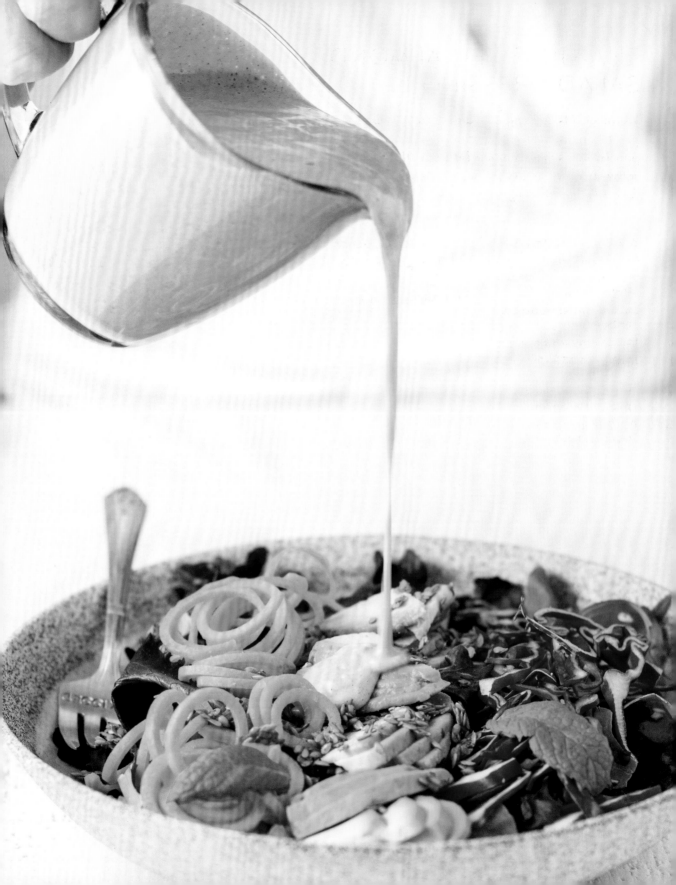

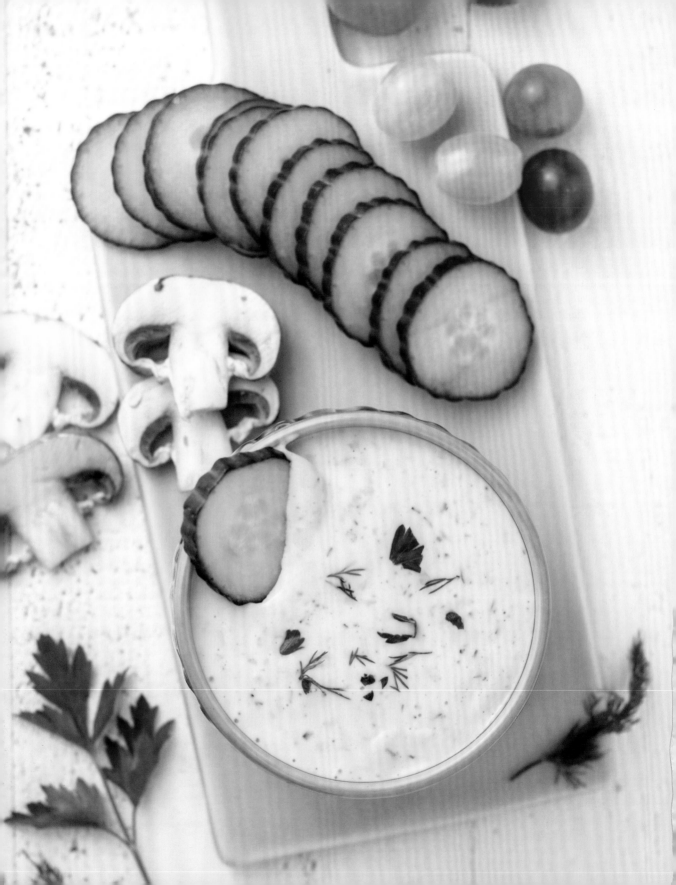

COCONUT RANCH DRESSING

Save money and get the most nutrition from your salad dressing by making it yourself. Ranch dressing is mostly oil, so store-bought versions made with refined oils are not ideal. This version incorporates a quick homemade mayo and is kept dairy-free using coconut milk, which adds a lightly sweet flavor.

1 large egg

1 tablespoon (15 ml) fresh lemon juice

2 teaspoons Dijon mustard

½ teaspoon sea salt

¾ cup (180 ml) avocado oil

¼ cup (60 ml) full-fat coconut milk, plus more as needed

¼ cup (15 g) chopped Italian parsley

2 tablespoons (8 g) chopped fresh dill

1 garlic clove, chopped

½ teaspoon onion powder

Black pepper to taste

In a blender, combine the egg, lemon juice, Dijon, and salt. Process to combine. With the blender running, slowly drizzle in the oil. This process should take at least 30 seconds, and by the time it's finished, a thick creamy mayo will form.

To the mayo in the blender, add the remaining ingredients. Use a spatula to stir the coconut milk into the mayo for easier blending. Process for about 1 minute to mix the ingredients fully. Thin with more coconut milk, if desired. Chill before serving.

Refrigerate leftovers in an airtight container for up to 1 week.

NOTE

Look for pastured eggs for this recipe. Conventionally raised eggs are at a much higher risk of carrying salmonella, which is the reason we are cautioned against consuming raw eggs. Because pastured chickens aren't packed into concentrated feeding lots, the risk of disease is much lower. One tip is to wash pastured eggs before consuming them raw; if salmonella is present, it will be on the shell.

YIELD

10 SERVINGS

NUTRITIONAL ANALYSIS

PER SERVING (2 TABLESPOONS, OR 30 ML):

164 CALORIES

18G FAT

1G PROTEIN

1G CARBOHYDRATE

1G DIETARY FIBER

MANGO-TARRAGON DRESSING

Sweet mango makes a satisfying and unique base for this low-calorie dressing. I love this dressing drizzled on seafood and greens as a simple delicious meal. I keep organic mango chunks in the freezer and toss them directly into the blender when the mood strikes. Fresh mango works as well.

¾ cup (135 g) mango chunks

2 tablespoons (30 ml) olive oil

2 tablespoons (30 ml) red wine vinegar

1 tablespoon (15 ml) fresh lemon juice

2 tablespoons (8 g) chopped fresh tarragon

Sea salt and black pepper to taste

In a blender, combine all the dressing ingredients and process until smooth. Taste and season with salt and pepper, as needed.

Refrigerate in an airtight container for up to 10 days.

YIELD

8 SERVINGS

NUTRITIONAL ANALYSIS

PER SERVING (2 TABLESPOONS, OR 30 ML):

47 CALORIES

4G FAT

1G PROTEIN

3G CARBOHYDRATE

1G DIETARY FIBER

ADD IT!

I love tarragon, and this dressing is the perfect opportunity to use it. However, when I'm without it, I use cilantro and Italian parsley in its place. Fresh basil would also pair wonderfully with this sweet, tangy dressing.

CHAPTER 8

◆ ◆ ◆

DESSERT

Life is too short to not enjoy sweet treats. The desserts here contain nutritious, whole food ingredients, and are lightly sweetened with natural, lower glycemic sweeteners.

Although healthier, these desserts are meant to be occasional treats. Diabetics or those who struggle with weight maintenance might want to avoid desserts or save them for special occasions. Some of the recipes in this chapter can be adapted to use with monk fruit or stevia, further lowering the glycemic load.

DARK CHOCOLATE–RASPBERRY SHORTBREAD BARS

It will be hard to believe this rich, decadent dessert is made from wholesome ingredients. A buttery almond flour shortbread is topped with a chewy chocolate-date layer, raspberries, and a drizzle of antioxidant-rich dark chocolate. Life is not worth living without splurging on healthy treats once in a while.

FOR SHORTBREAD:

6 tablespoons (¾ stick; 84 g) pastured butter, at room temperature

¼ cup (80 g) honey

½ teaspoon vanilla extract

2 cups (193 g) blanched almond flour

Pinch sea salt

FOR CHOCOLATE-DATE LAYER:

20 ounces (560 g) pitted Medjool dates

¼ cup (22 g) cacao powder

3 tablespoons (42 g) pastured butter, at room temperature

Pinch sea salt

FOR TOPPING:

1 cup (125 g) fresh raspberries

1¾ ounces (50 g) 85% or 100% dark chocolate, melted

YIELD

16 SERVINGS

NUTRITIONAL ANALYSIS

PER SERVING (1 BAR):

287 CALORIES

15G FAT

5G PROTEIN

40G CARBOHYDRATE

6G DIETARY FIBER

To make the shortbread: Preheat the oven to 350°F (180°C, or gas mark 4). Line an 8 × 8-inch (20 × 20 cm) baking pan with parchment paper.

In the bowl of a stand mixer fitted with the paddle attachment, or in a large bowl and using a hand mixer, beat the butter, honey, and vanilla on medium speed until light and fluffy.

Add the almond flour and salt (up to ¼ teaspoon if the butter is unsalted) and mix until there is no dry flour left.

Press the shortbread dough into the prepared pan. Use a pastry roller, or your hands, to flatten the dough into a smooth and even layer. Use a fork or a chopstick to poke holes across the shortbread to ensure the dough cooks in the center as well as around the edges.

Bake the shortbread for 22 to 24 minutes until the top is a light golden brown. Remove from the oven and let cool fully before topping with the chocolate-date layer.

To make the chocolate-date layer: Place the dates in a medium-size bowl and cover them with boiling water. Let soak for about 5 minutes. Drain all the water from the dates and transfer to a food processor.

Add the cacao powder, butter, and salt. Process for 3 to 4 minutes, stopping to scrape the mixture from the sides about every minute or so. The mixture is ready when there are no pieces of date visible and the mixture is smooth and caramel-like. If necessary, add 1 to 2 tablespoons (15 to 30 ml) of hot water to reach the desired texture.

Once the shortbread has fully cooled, spread the chocolate-date mixture over the top and use wet hands to flatten it into a smooth layer.

To make the topping: Top the date layer with the raspberries and drizzle with the melted dark chocolate. Chill thoroughly before cutting and serving.

Refrigerate leftovers tightly wrapped, or in an airtight container, for up to 4 days.

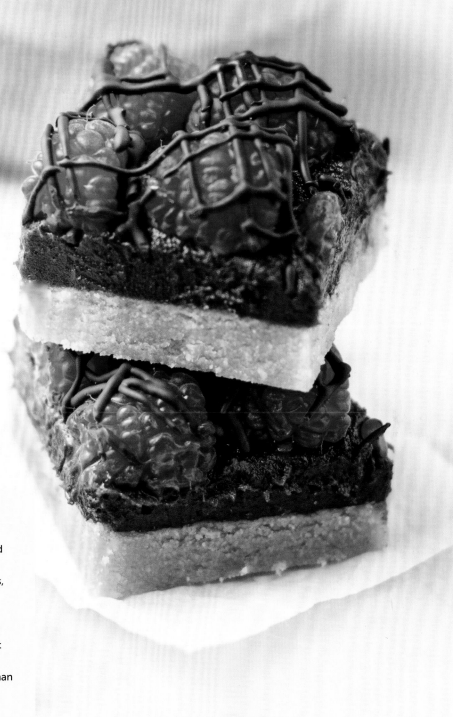

MAPLE-PECAN MACAROONS

Macaroons are very easy to make and always taste like a special treat. This version uses maple syrup as a sweetener, which adds a delicious rich flavor that complements the pecans. Because these cookies are sweet on their own, I use an unsweetened chocolate for dipping and drizzling the cookies.

3 large egg whites

⅓ cup (107 g) maple syrup

1 teaspoon grass-fed gelatin

½ teaspoon almond exact

½ teaspoon vanilla extract

2 cups (170 g) finely shredded unsweetened coconut

½ cup (55 g) finely chopped pecans, plus more for garnish (optional)

3 ounces (85 g) unsweetened chocolate

Preheat the oven to 350°F (180°C, or gas mark 4). Line a baking sheet with parchment paper or a silicone baking mat.

In a medium-size bowl, whisk the egg whites and maple syrup until very foamy. It isn't necessary to whisk to form peaks, like in a meringue, but the mixture should be lightened.

Add the gelatin, almond extract, and vanilla and whisk well.

Add the coconut and pecans and stir to evenly coat with the egg white mixture.

Use a rounded tablespoon or cookie scoop to scoop and compact the coconut batter, pressing it to hold it together well, before placing it on the prepared baking sheet. Repeat to make 20 cookies.

Bake the cookies for 16 to 18 minutes until lightly browned on top. Let cool fully.

In a double boiler, melt the unsweetened chocolate. Dip the base of each cookie into the melted chocolate to coat, placing them on a piece of wax paper to set. Use a fork to drizzle any remaining chocolate on the tops of the cookies. Sprinkle the cookies with additional chopped pecans (if using).

YIELD

20 SERVINGS

NUTRITIONAL ANALYSIS

PER SERVING (1 COOKIE):

85 CALORIES

7G FAT

2G PROTEIN

6G CARBOHYDRATE

2G DIETARY FIBER

NOTE

If using unsweetened chocolate as a coating sounds strange to you, try it before discounting it. The sweetness of the cookie is enough to lighten the flavor of the chocolate.

ADD IT!

Macaroons are a great gluten-free nutrient-dense cookie. This recipe can be made without the nuts, or using another nut, such as sliced almonds or chopped walnuts. The chocolate coating is another optional (though delicious!) ingredient.

SUPERFOODS DARK CHOCOLATE BARK

Keeping a stash of this easy-to-make treat in the refrigerator will make sure you turn to something packed with antioxidants when those sweet cravings hit. Dark chocolate and pomegranate are both nutritional powerhouses and a delicious combination, especially when sprinkled with lots of crunchy nuts and seeds. I use a combination of pumpkin seeds, pecans, and hemp seeds here, but experiment with your favorites.

6 ounces (170 g) 85% or higher dark chocolate

1 tablespoon (14 g) coconut oil

½ cup (90 g) pomegranate arils, divided

2 tablespoons (14 g) chopped pecans

2 tablespoons (16 g) pumpkin seeds

1 tablespoon (10 g) hemp seeds

Line a small baking sheet with parchment paper. Set aside.

In a double boiler, melt the chocolate and coconut oil, stirring until the mixture is smooth and fully melted. Stir in ¼ cup (45 g) of the pomegranate arils. Pour the chocolate mixture onto the prepared baking sheet and spread into a large rectangle.

Sprinkle the top of the chocolate with the remaining ¼ cup (45 g) of pomegranate arils, as well as the pecans and seeds.

Refrigerate for about 20 minutes to set the chocolate, then break it into smaller pieces.

Keep refrigerated in an airtight container for about 1 week, or freeze for up to 3 months. Enjoy right out of the freezer to keep from melting.

YIELD

12 SERVINGS

NUTRITIONAL ANALYSIS

PER SERVING (1/12 OF RECIPE):

131 CALORIES

10G FAT

2G PROTEIN

9G CARBOHYDRATE

2G DIETARY FIBER

ADD IT!

Chocolate can be loaded with sugar. Look for 85 to 90 percent dark chocolate, or opt for one that's sweetened with coconut sugar or monk fruit. The pomegranate arils add pops of sweetness.

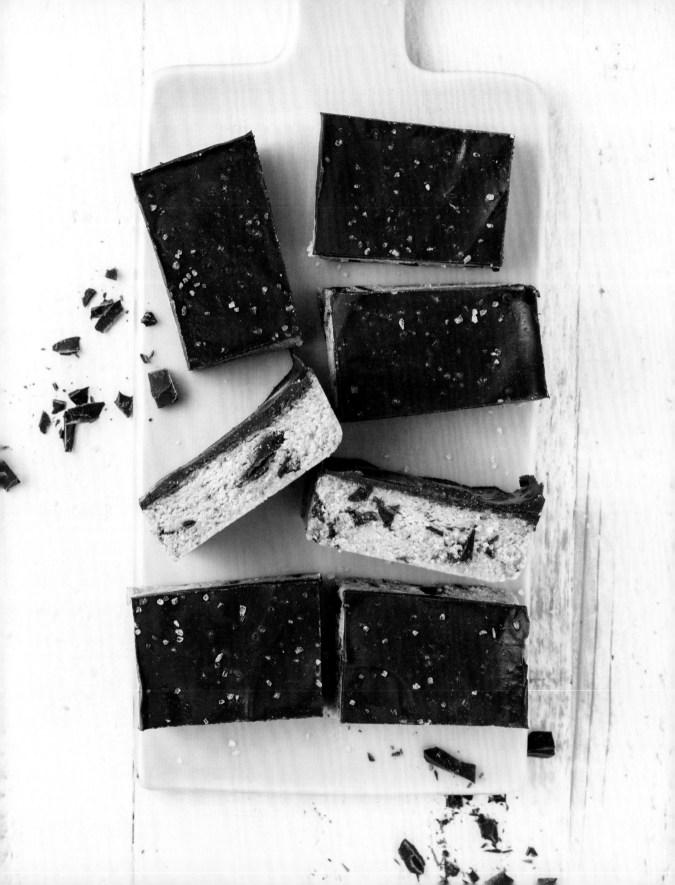

NO-BAKE COOKIE DOUGH BARS

A simple no-bake cookie recipe for days that chocolate is a must. I like to cut these into small squares and keep these high-energy treats in the freezer for on-the-go energy boosts. Nutrient-dense cashews and buckwheat form the base of these healthy bars. Choose 80 to 90 percent dark chocolate for the most health benefits, or look for bars sweetened with monk fruit or stevia. Recipe inspired by fitmittenkitchen.com.

FOR COOKIE DOUGH:

¾ cup (90 g) raw buckwheat groats

1 cup (260 g) cashew butter

¼ cup (80 g) maple syrup

2 tablespoons (28 g) coconut oil, melted

½ teaspoon sea salt

1 vanilla bean, scraped (reserve the pod for another use, like in smoothies)

1½ ounces (42 g) 85% to 90% dark chocolate, chopped

Coarse sea salt, for garnish (optional)

FOR CASHEW FUDGE:

2 tablespoons (33 g) cashew butter

1½ ounces (42 g) 85% to 90% dark chocolate, chopped

Line a standard loaf pan with parchment paper. Set aside.

To make the cookie dough: In a blender, process the buckwheat groats into a fine flour. Set aside.

In a medium-size bowl, combine the cashew butter, maple syrup, melted coconut oil, sea salt, and scraped vanilla bean seeds. Stir the ingredients well to combine.

Add the buckwheat flour and dark chocolate. Stir to combine until no dry flour remains. Press the cookie dough into the prepared loaf pan in an even layer.

To make the cashew fudge: In a small saucepan over very low heat, or in a double boiler, combine the cashew butter and dark chocolate. Cook for about 5 minutes, stirring to mix the ingredients until fully melted, being careful not to scorch the chocolate. Spread the fudge over the cookie dough in an even layer. Sprinkle with coarse sea salt (if using).

Freeze the cookie dough bars for 30 minutes to set. Remove the bars from the freezer and cut into slices. To cut the bars without the chocolate cracking, let them sit at room temperature for 10 minutes to soften the fudge layer before cutting into them.

YIELD

18 SERVINGS

NUTRITIONAL ANALYSIS

PER SERVING (1 BAR):

160 CALORIES

15G FAT

4G PROTEIN

12G CARBOHYDRATE

2G DIETARY FIBER

NOTE

The coconut oil helps hold these bars together when they are chilled.

NOTE

Make these bars grain-free and lower the carbs by using ground almonds instead of buckwheat groats. Substitute ¾ cup (110 g) whole almonds. Process them in a blender until a flour forms, being careful not to overprocess into a butter.

ALMOND BERRY COBBLER

This delicious summery dessert is just about too good to be true. Once you've tried this recipe, you'll realize how unnecessary the typical cup-plus of sugar is when added to fruit-based desserts.

FOR BERRY FILLING:

8 cups (1.2 kg) fresh mixed berries (I used 3 cups strawberries, 3 cups blueberries, and 2 cups blackberries)

2 tablespoons (16 g) arrowroot

1 tablespoon (20 g) maple syrup

1 teaspoon fresh lemon juice

1 vanilla bean, scraped (reserve the pod for another use, like in smoothies)

FOR BISCUIT TOPPING:

¼ cup (60 ml) unsweetened Almond Milk (page 173) or store-bought almond milk

¼ cup (56 g) coconut oil, melted

3 tablespoons (60 g) maple syrup

½ teaspoon almond extract

½ teaspoon sea salt

½ teaspoon baking soda

2 cups (192 g) blanched almond flour

¼ cup (32 g) arrowroot

1 large egg white, beaten (optional)

⅓ cup (31 g) raw sliced almonds

YIELD

9 SERVINGS

NUTRITIONAL ANALYSIS

PER SERVING (¾ CUP, OR 163 G):

294 CALORIES

19G FAT

6G PROTEIN

30G CARBOHYDRATE

7G DIETARY FIBER

Preheat the oven to 400°F (200°C, or gas mark 6).

To make the berry filling: In a large bowl, combine the berries, arrowroot, maple syrup, lemon juice, and scraped vanilla bean seeds. Gently mix to coat the berries evenly. Transfer to an 8 x 8-inch (20 x 20 cm) baking dish.

To make the biscuit topping: In a medium-size bowl, whisk the almond milk, melted coconut oil, maple syrup, and almond extract to combine. Add the salt and baking soda and whisk again to incorporate.

Add the almond flour and arrowroot and use a spoon to mix the dry ingredients into the wet ingredients, until no dry ingredients remain. Spoon the biscuit topping over the berries in 3 rows of 3 mounds. Use the spoon to gently mix up the topping and spread it over the top, making a rustic, uneven covering.

Brush the biscuits with the beaten egg white to make a beautiful shiny topping (if using).

Evenly sprinkle the almonds over the topping. Cover the baking dish with aluminum foil.

Bake the cobbler for 35 minutes, covered. Remove the foil and bake the cobbler for 12 to 15 minutes more until the topping is lightly browned. Almond flour browns and burns quickly, so check on the cobbler before the end of the baking time.

Refrigerate leftovers tightly wrapped, or in an airtight container, for up to 4 days.

NOTE

If using frozen berries, prepare the berry filling and let it sit at room temperature for 30 minutes to 1 hour to thaw before topping and baking the cobbler. The cobbler topping won't bake with frozen berries.

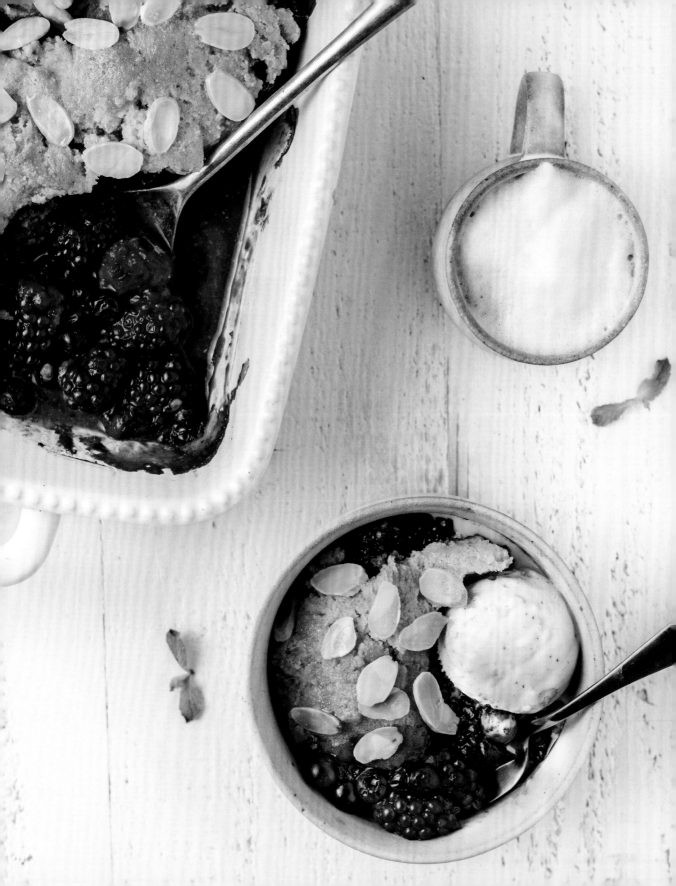

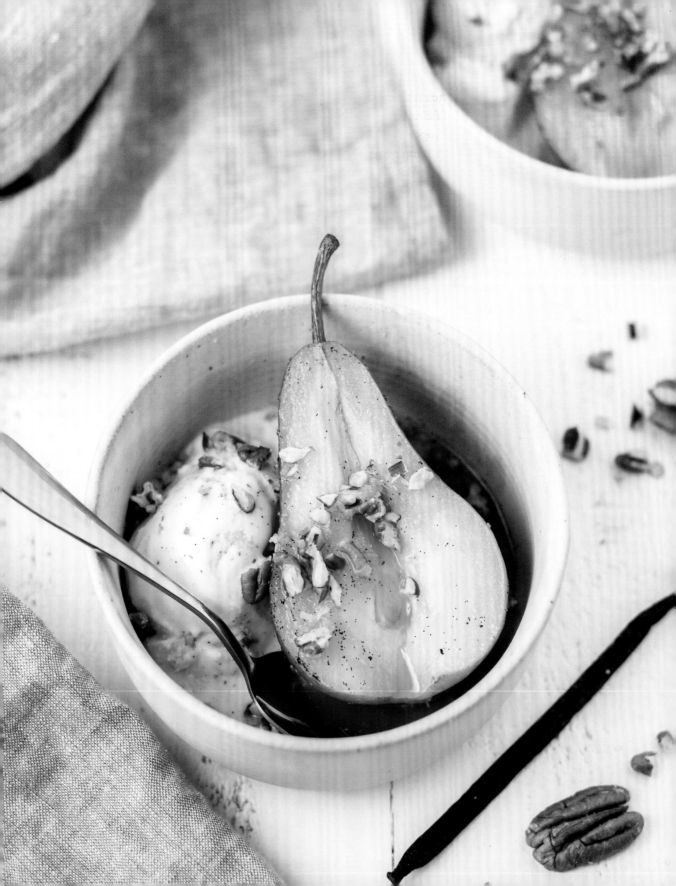

VANILLA-POACHED PEARS

A ripe, sweet pear on its own has a creamy, dessertlike taste. This recipe gently cooks the fruit in a vanilla- and cinnamon-spiked white wine sauce. The standard French recipe calls for a thick sugar syrup, but you'll find that just a touch of maple syrup in the wine is more than sufficient and lets the pears shine. Serve these pears warm over a scoop of Vanilla Bean Coconut Milk Custard (page 168).

2 firm pears, any variety

1 vanilla bean

1½ cups (360 ml) water

1 cup (240 ml) sweet white wine, such as Moscato

1 tablespoon (20 g) maple syrup

1 tablespoon (15 ml) fresh lemon juice

1 cinnamon stick

1 teaspoon grated lemon zest

¼ cup (28 g) chopped pecans

Halve the pears and cut out the core and seeds. Leave the stem on the pears for presentation, if desired.

Halve the vanilla bean lengthwise so the seeds are exposed.

In a small skillet large enough to hold the pears in a single layer, over medium heat, arrange the pears halves and add the water, white wine, maple syrup, lemon juice, vanilla bean, cinnamon stick, and lemon zest. Bring to a simmer.

Cover the skillet and cook for 7 minutes. Remove the lid, flip the pears, and simmer for 7 minutes more to concentrate the syrup until it is reduced to about ½ cup (120 ml). If the syrup becomes too concentrated, thin it with a few tablespoons (about 45 ml) of water.

Serve the pears with a drizzle of the white wine syrup, topped with 1 tablespoon (7 g) of chopped pecans.

YIELD

4 SERVINGS

NUTRITIONAL ANALYSIS

PER SERVING (½ PEAR, 2 TABLESPOONS, OR 30 ML, SYRUP, AND 1 TABLESPOON, OR 7 G, CHOPPED PECANS):

160 CALORIES

5G FAT

1G PROTEIN

20G CARBOHYDRATE

3G DIETARY FIBER

NOTE

Alcohol evaporates when cooked, so this recipe is suitable for children. Make this recipe alcohol-free by using ¾ cup (180 ml) apple juice along with ¾ cup (180 ml) water in place of the sweet wine.

TROPICAL PANNA COTTA

This gelatin-based dessert is lightly sweet and the perfect way to end a summer meal. Coconut milk is lightly spiced and served with a tropical fruit topping. I use a silicone mini cheesecake mold to make perfectly portioned desserts. These can also be made and served in ramekins.

FOR PANNA COTTA:

2 cups (480 ml) full-fat coconut milk, divided

2 teaspoons grass-fed gelatin

1 tablespoon (20 g) raw honey

1 cinnamon stick

½ vanilla bean

¼ teaspoon ground ginger

FOR FRUIT TOPPING:

½ cup (90 g) diced fresh mango

½ cup (90 g) diced fresh papaya

1 tablespoon (8 g) unsweetened shredded coconut

1 tablespoon (15 ml) fresh lime juice

To make the panna cotta: In a small saucepan, whisk ¼ cup (60 ml) of the coconut milk and the gelatin to combine. Let sit for 1 to 2 minutes to bloom and absorb some water.

Add the remaining 1¾ cups (420 ml) of coconut milk and the remaining panna cotta ingredients to the saucepan and whisk to combine. Heat the mixture over medium heat, whisking often, until it begins to boil. Boil for 1 minute, then remove from the heat. Remove and discard the cinnamon stick and vanilla bean.

Pour the panna cotta mixture into a silicone mold or silicone muffin liners. Refrigerate for at least 2 hours to set.

To make the fruit topping: In a small bowl, stir together the fruit, coconut, and lime juice.

To serve, unmold the panna cotta and top with the tropical fruit topping.

YIELD

4 SERVINGS

NUTRITIONAL ANALYSIS

PER SERVING (1 PANNA COTTA AND ¼ CUP, OR 45 G, FRUIT TOPPING):

270 CALORIES

15G FAT

4G PROTEIN

13G CARBOHYDRATE

1G DIETARY FIBER

NOTE

Coconut milk is naturally sweet, meaning this easy dessert needs very little added sweetener. This recipe adapts well to using noncaloric sweeteners like monk fruit and stevia.

ADD IT!

Mixed berries are another great topping for this dessert. Try a mix of blackberries, raspberries, and blueberries for a cooling summer treat.

CHERRY COCONUT SORBET

Here's a sweet summertime treat that can be ready in an instant (almost!). Keeping frozen cherries and coconut milk on hand is easy to do and processing this two-ingredient dessert into a dreamy, creamy sorbet takes just minutes.

3 cups (465 g) frozen cherries

½ cup (120 ml) coconut milk

In a high-speed blender or food processor, combine the cherries and coconut milk. Process on high speed until smooth and creamy. It helps to use a blender with a tamper stick, or to stop the food processor and scrape down the sides a few times throughout the process.

The dessert is a soft-serve consistency and delicious served right away. If you'd like to serve this sorbet in scoops, transfer it to a shallow container, cover, and freeze for 1 to 2 hours.

Freeze leftovers in an ice-cube tray, then store the sorbet cubes in an airtight container. Let the cubes thaw slightly for 10 to 15 minutes before putting them into the food processor to re-blend into a creamy dessert.

YIELD

4 SERVINGS

NUTRITIONAL ANALYSIS

PER SERVING (⅔ CUP, OR 140 G):

121 CALORIES

6G FAT

2G PROTEIN

17G CARBOHYDRATE

2G DIETARY FIBER

NOTE

Fruit is a great dessert option on the pegan diet, but it should be enjoyed in moderation. People with diabetes or people who struggle with weight loss might want to choose desserts made with low glycemic index fruits (see page 11).

ADD IT!

This simple recipe is perfect for fruit higher in sugar, such as pineapple, mango, and bananas. It also works with red dragon fruit. Omit the cherries and substitute 1½ cups (weight varies) of your fruit of choice.

VANILLA BEAN COCONUT MILK CUSTARD

This dairy-free frozen custard is the perfect complement to the Almond Berry Cobbler (page 162) or Vanilla-Poached Pears (page 165) and a wonderful treat drizzled with Cashew Hot Fudge (page 170). As with most homemade ice creams, this is best served within a couple hours of making it.

6 large egg yolks

2 tablespoons (40 g) maple syrup

2¼ cups (540 ml) coconut milk

⅛ teaspoon sea salt

1 vanilla bean, scraped (reserve the pod for another use, like in smoothies)

In a medium-size saucepan over medium heat, whisk the egg yolks and maple syrup to combine. Whisk in the coconut milk.

Gently cook the mixture for about 10 minutes, whisking occasionally, or until the custard reaches 170°F (77°C).

Whisk in the salt and scraped vanilla bean seeds. Let the custard cool. Refrigerate until chilled.

Transfer the chilled custard to an ice-cream maker and freeze according to the manufacturer's instructions.

Enjoy right out of the ice-cream maker or add to a shallow storage container and freeze for 1 to 2 hours for a scoopable ice cream.

YIELD

5 SERVINGS

NUTRITIONAL ANALYSIS

PER SERVING (½ CUP, OR ABOUT 100 G):

243 CALORIES

23G FAT

5G PROTEIN

8G CARBOHYDRATE

6G DIETARY FIBER

NOTE

Rather than tossing the egg whites, set them aside and make a batch of Maple-Pecan Macaroons (page 158) to keep in the freezer for sweet snacking later on.

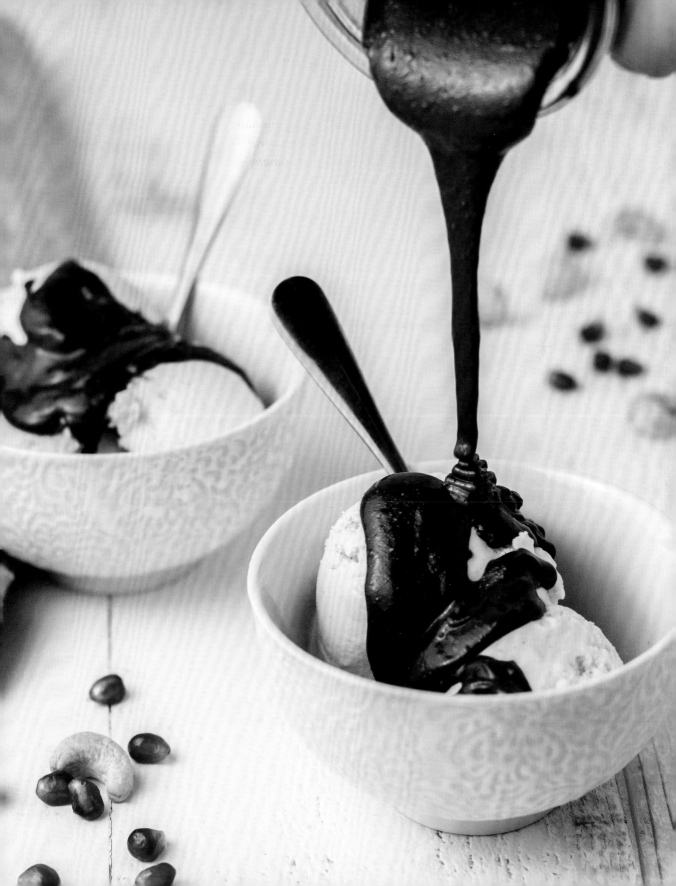

CASHEW HOT FUDGE

Even something as sinful as hot fudge can be recreated with pegan diet–approved ingredients. This thick, creamy, rich chocolate sauce is perfect for drizzling on Vanilla Bean Coconut Milk Custard (page 168) or Cherry Coconut Sorbet (page 167). So good, you'll never be tempted to buy standard chocolate sauce again.

6 tablespoons (98 g) cashew butter

6 tablespoons (30 g) cacao powder (see note)

3 tablespoons (45 ml) avocado oil

2 tablespoons (28 g) coconut oil

2 tablespoons (40 g) maple syrup or date syrup

Pinch sea salt

In a small saucepan, whisk all the ingredients to combine well. If your coconut oil is solid, don't worry. It will melt into the sauce in the next step.

Place the saucepan over low heat, and cook, whisking, for about 5 minutes until the sauce is melted, warmed, and easily whisks together. It does not need to bubble.

Store leftovers at room temperature. The sauce will thicken when it cools, so reheat it before using again. I like to store it in a glass jar and put the glass jar in hot water for 5 to 10 minutes, stirring it well halfway through the heating time. If necessary, thin it with more coconut oil.

YIELD

7 SERVINGS

NUTRITIONAL ANALYSIS

PER SERVING (2 TABLESPOONS, OR 30 ML):

196 CALORIES

18G FAT

3G PROTEIN

10G CARBOHYDRATE

2G DIETARY FIBER

NOTE

Cacao powder is ground-up cacao nibs processed at low heat with the cocoa butter and most of the nutrients still intact. The fats in cacao beans are monounsaturated and heart healthy. This gives the sauce a richer flavor. A natural cocoa powder will work as a substitution but does not yield the same health benefits.

CHAPTER 9

DRINKS

The best drinks on a pegan diet are water, coffee, and tea. Many common beverages are loaded with sugar and cause spikes in blood sugar levels without offering nutritional value. Some exceptions are unsweetened nut milks, vegetable juices, and smoothies made with low glycemic index foods. Make these drinks at home to control the quality of the ingredients used in your beverages.

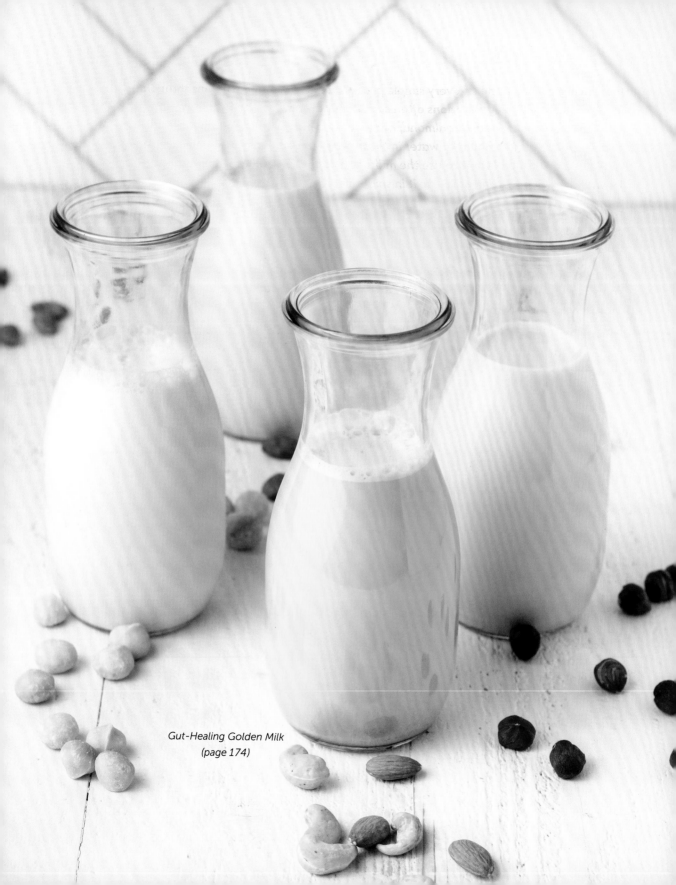

Gut-Healing Golden Milk
(page 174)

NUT MILKS

Making nut milk at home is a very simple process and the freshness comes through in the taste. Store-bought options often contain sugars and gums. You can make milk from any nut or seed, but almond, hazelnut, and macadamia nut are my favorites. Adjust the amount of water in these recipes to suit your preference. I use less water when I want to use the milks as a coffee creamer, and more when I want nut milk for a drink or to use it in smoothies.

FOR ALMOND MILK:

1 cup (145 g) almonds

2 to 4 cups (480 to 960 ml) water

FOR HAZELNUT MILK:

1 cup (135 g) hazelnuts

2 to 4 cups (480 to 960 ml) water

FOR MACADAMIA NUT MILK:

1 cup (135 g) macadamia nuts

2 to 4 cups (480 to 960 ml) water

ADD IT!

Vanilla beans and Medjool dates are often added to flavor homemade nut milks. Add 1 vanilla bean and, optionally, 1 or 2 pitted Medjool dates to the blender and process with the nuts and water for a sweet vanilla nut milk, which is particularly nice if you're making a coffee creamer.

YIELD

3 SERVINGS

NUTRITIONAL ANALYSIS

FOR ALMOND MILK (UNSWEETENED)
PER SERVING (1 CUP, OR 240 ML):

30 CALORIES

2.5G FAT

1G PROTEIN

1G CARBOHYDRATE

1G DIETARY FIBER

FOR HAZELNUT MILK (UNSWEETENED)
PER SERVING (1 CUP, OR 240 ML):

70 CALORIES

4G FAT

3G PROTEIN

1G CARBOHYDRATE

1G DIETARY FIBER

FOR MACADAMIA NUT MILK (UNSWEETENED)
PER SERVING (1 CUP, OR 240 ML):

50 CALORIES

4G FAT

1G PROTEIN

1G CARBOHYDRATE

1G DIETARY FIBER

Soak the almonds, hazelnuts, or macadamia nuts in water overnight, or up to 24 hours. Drain and rinse the nuts, then transfer to a high-speed blender.

Add 2 cups (480 ml) of water for a thick nut cream, good for coffee creamer. Add 4 cups (960 ml) of water for a thinner beverage, good for drinking or adding to smoothies.

Process on high speed for 1 to 2 minutes until the nuts are fully broken down and the liquid is thick and white.

Drain the nut milk through cheesecloth lining a bowl, or in a nut milk bag set over a bowl.

Refrigerate fresh nut milk in an airtight container for 3 to 4 days. Because they do not contain additives, fresh nut milks do not last as long as store-bought versions.

GUT-HEALING GOLDEN MILK

Turmeric and ginger have powerful anti-inflammatory properties and, combined, are used to relieve pain, decrease nausea, and enhance immune function. This delicious spiced nut milk is wonderful warmed or served over ice. The method requires soaking the nuts overnight, so plan accordingly.

½ cup (73 g) almonds

½ cup (70 g) cashews

3 cups (720 ml) water

1 Medjool date, pitted, or 2 tablespoons (18 g) date sugar

1 tablespoon (6 g) sliced peeled fresh ginger

½ teaspoon ground turmeric

¼ teaspoon ground cinnamon

½ vanilla bean, scraped (reserve the pod for another use, like in smoothies)

Soak the almonds and cashews in water overnight.

Drain and rinse the nuts, then add them to a high-speed blender along with the remaining ingredients. Blend well, for 1 to 2 minutes, until the nuts are broken down into a pulp.

Drain the nut milk through cheesecloth lining a bowl, or in a nut milk bag set over a bowl. Serve chilled or warmed.

Fresh nut milks sour quickly. Refrigerate leftovers in an airtight container for up to 3 days.

YIELD

3 SERVINGS

NUTRITIONAL ANALYSIS

PER SERVING (1 CUP, OR 240 ML):

71 CALORIES

4G FAT

2G PROTEIN

8G CARBOHYDRATE

1G DIETARY FIBER

NOTE

Date sugar is made from grinding whole dates, so the nutrition is very similar to using whole dried dates. It's easy to keep on hand and easier to strain when making nut milks. If you regularly sweeten your nut milk, buy a bag for your convenience.

METABOLISM-BOOSTING REFRESHER

Grapefruit has an antioxidant called naringenin that is known for helping your body process insulin more effectively, which aids with weight loss. One grapefruit is enough to enjoy this effect, so keep the sugar level down in your drink by combining it with water-rich green vegetables. You'll be surprised at how sweet this juice is, even though only a small portion is fruit juice.

1 grapefruit, peeled

½ **cucumber**

½ **zucchini**

2 celery stalks

Run all the ingredients through a juicer and enjoy cold or over ice.

YIELD

1 SERVING

NUTRITIONAL ANALYSIS

PER SERVING (12 OUNCES, OR 360 ML):

67 CALORIES

0G FAT

3G PROTEIN

18G CARBOHYDRATE

1G DIETARY FIBER

NOTE

Juicing is not the best habit for weight loss. However, when you're feeling the need for a burst of nutrients, a mixture of low glycemic index fruits and lots of veggies gives you a hydrating energy boost.

MUSCLE-RECOVERY JUICE

Restore your electrolytes naturally with this refreshing vegetable juice. Beets are an excellent source of dietary nitrates, which your body converts into nitric oxide, a compound that helps with faster muscle recovery and reduced inflammation. Combine that with potassium-rich beet greens and this juice is the perfect recipe for making you feel better in the morning.

1 fresh beet

2 beet greens

1 cucumber

2 celery stalks

½ lemon, peeled

Run all the ingredients through a juicer and enjoy cold or over ice.

YIELD

1 SERVING

NUTRITIONAL ANALYSIS

PER SERVING (12 OUNCES, OR 360 ML):

59 CALORIES

0G FAT

4G PROTEIN

18G CARBOHYDRATE

1G DIETARY FIBER

NOTE

Reserve juicing for very active days, especially if you're diabetic or trying to lose weight.

VANILLA MATCHA SMOOTHIE

If you're a green tea ice-cream fan, this smoothie is for you. It's energizing, nourishing, and super creamy. Instead of using nut milk, this recipe calls for cashew butter, which is easy to keep on hand and makes a rich, smooth base. Using frozen cauliflower and spinach adds fiber and nutrients while keeping the overall sugar content low.

1½ bananas, quartered and frozen

1 cup (132 g) frozen cauliflower florets

2 cups (60 g) fresh spinach

2 cups (480 ml) water

2 tablespoons (32 g) cashew butter

2 teaspoons matcha green tea

½ vanilla bean pod (see note)

In a high-speed blender, combine all the ingredients and process until a very thick and creamy smoothie forms.

YIELD

2 SERVINGS

NUTRITIONAL ANALYSIS

PER SERVING (10 OUNCES, OR 285 ML):

210 CALORIES

9G FAT

8G PROTEIN

29G CARBOHYDRATE

4G DIETARY FIBER

NOTE

When I use just the inside seeds of a vanilla bean, like in the Tropical Panna Cotta (page 166), I save the vanilla bean pods to use in smoothies like this one. The pods burst with flavor and blend well into smoothies.

ADD IT!

If you don't have cauliflower, use another veggie, like frozen zucchini, in its place. I like to toss cauliflower and zucchini into the freezer when I know I won't use it before it goes bad, then toss into smoothies instead of ice to keep them thick and icy.

AVOCADO-MINT CHIP SMOOTHIE

Like your favorite ice cream flavor but packed with superfoods, this lower-carb smoothie is a great sweet treat.

2 bananas, quartered and frozen

½ avocado, pitted and flesh scooped from the peel

1 cup (30 g) fresh spinach

¾ cup (180 ml) Almond Milk (page 173) or other store-bought plant-based milk

¼ cup (60 ml) coconut milk

½ to ¾ teaspoon peppermint extract

½ teaspoon vanilla extract

½ cup (60 g) ice cubes

½ ounce (14 g) 100% dark chocolate, roughly chopped

In a high speed blender, combine the bananas, avocado, spinach, almond milk, coconut milk, peppermint extract, vanilla, and ice. Process on high speed until very thick and smooth. The spinach should color the smoothie green but be completely broken down and indiscernible.

Add the chocolate and pulse a few times to break it down. Leave some texture to the chocolate so it's similar to having chocolate chips in your smoothie.

YIELD

2 SERVINGS

NUTRITIONAL ANALYSIS

PER SERVING (½ SMOOTHIE RECIPE):

287 CALORIES

15G FAT

5G PROTEIN

40G CARBOHYDRATE

6G DIETARY FIBER

NOTE

To keep this delicious smoothie a "milk shake" consistency, be sure to use frozen bananas and add ice. I also keep spinach in the freezer so I always have it on hand. The coconut milk adds richness and sweetness, so I don't recommend swapping it out.

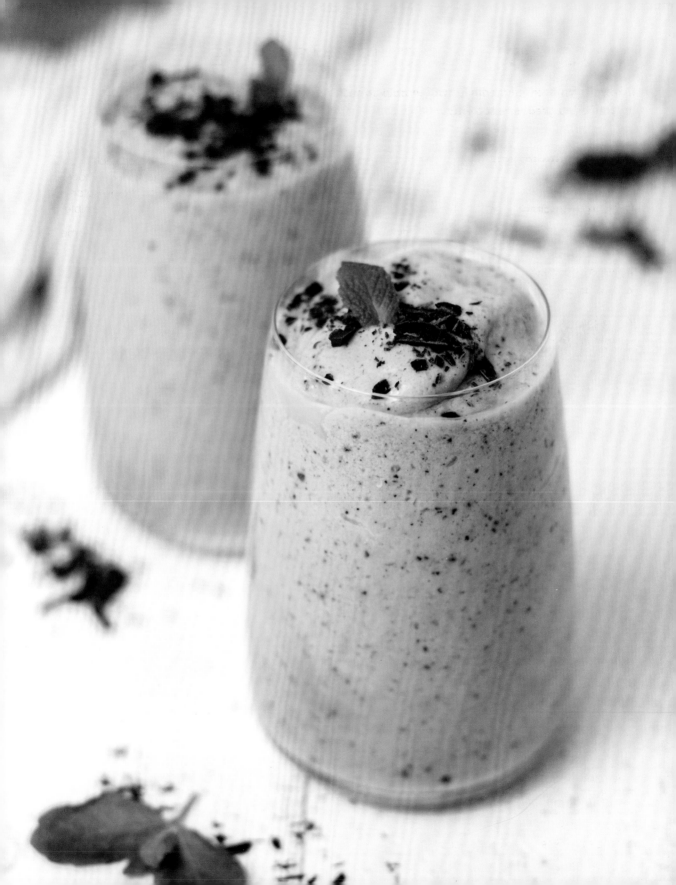

LEMON-BLUEBERRY SMOOTHIE

This nourishing smoothie packs a flavor punch. Blueberries and lemon are a match made in heaven and adding hemp seeds and spinach means more protein and fiber. Try unsweetened almond, oat, or cashew milk along with sweet and creamy coconut milk as a base. Using nut and coconut milks as a base reduces the amount of sugar in smoothies compared to options made with juice.

3 cups (90 g) fresh spinach

1½ cups (360 ml) unsweetened plant-based milk

½ cup (120 ml) full-fat coconut milk

1½ cups (233 g) frozen blueberries

1 banana, quartered and frozen

2 tablespoons (20 g) hemp seeds

1 tablespoon (15 ml) fresh lemon juice

1 teaspoon grated peeled fresh ginger (optional)

In a high-speed blender, combine all the ingredients and process until a thick and creamy smoothie forms.

YIELD

2 SERVINGS

NUTRITIONAL ANALYSIS

PER SERVING (1½ CUPS, OR 360 ML):

352 CALORIES

22G FAT

10G PROTEIN

35G CARBOHYDRATE

6G DIETARY FIBER

NOTE

If you find yourself looking to smoothies during the summer months for meal replacements, keep your freezer stocked with low-sugar berries and avocados and vegetables such as spinach, cauliflower, and zucchini.

ADD IT!

Try this smoothie with blackberries or raspberries in place of the blueberries. Both options are equally delicious with the creamy lemon flavor.

GOLDEN MILK HOT COCOA

The healing properties of ginger and turmeric are the perfect addition to a creamy mug of hot cocoa. It's a perfect sweet treat to end a cold day, especially when you're feeling worn down or your body is in need of rejuvenation.

1 cup Gut-Healing Golden Milk (page 174)

1 tablespoon (5 g) cacao powder

Monk fruit or stevia sweetener, to taste (optional)

In a small saucepan over medium heat, combine the golden milk and cacao. While gently warming the milk to your desired temperature, whisk to combine the cacao. Taste and adjust the sweetness with sweetener (if using).

NOTE

If you don't want to take the time to make Gut-Healing Golden Milk (page 174), substitute 1 cup (240 ml) nut-based milk, 1 tablespoon (10 g) date sugar, and a pinch each of ground turmeric, ground cinnamon, and ground ginger. It's also good sweetened with monk fruit or stevia in place of the date sugar.

YIELD

1 SERVING

NUTRITIONAL ANALYSIS

PER SERVING (1 CUP, OR 240 ML):

75 CALORIES

4G FAT

2G PROTEIN

9G CARBOHYDRATE

2G DIETARY FIBER

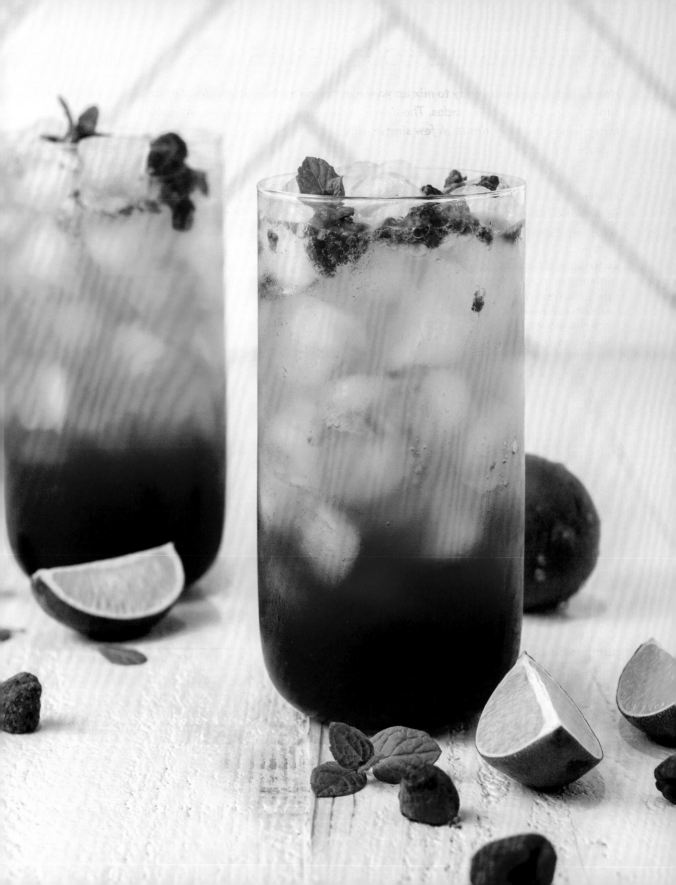

SPARKLING HIBISCUS REFRESHER

Herbal teas are a great way to mix up your hydration routine without turning to sugary drinks like juice or sodas. The deep hue of hibiscus tea is a good indicator that it's high in antioxidants. A few simple additions turn this tea into a craveable summer refresher.

4 bags hibiscus tea

1 cup (240 ml) boiling water

¼ cup (35 g) freeze-dried raspberries, crushed

2 tablespoons (30 ml) fresh lime juice

1 tablespoon (20 g) maple syrup, or monk fruit sweetener or stevia, to taste

1½ cups (360 ml) soda water

In a large glass measuring cup, combine the tea bags and boiling water. Steep the tea for 3 to 5 minutes. Remove and discard the bags and let the tea cool to room temperature.

Stir in the freeze-dried raspberries, lime juice, and maple syrup. Pour the tea mixture over ice and top with soda water.

YIELD

2 SERVINGS

NUTRITIONAL ANALYSIS

PER SERVING (1½ CUPS, OR 360 ML) USING MAPLE SYRUP:

50 CALORIES

1G FAT

1G PROTEIN

12G CARBOHYDRATE

1G DIETARY FIBER

NOTE

Try this simple recipe with any of your favorite teas. Green tea, ginger tea, and moringa tea all have beneficial health properties and are delicious in this recipe.

HAZELNUT LATTE

This homemade nut milk latte is the best treat on a cool morning. Use whatever coffee you enjoy. I make it with strong-brewed French press coffee, but espresso or a standard drip coffee work just as nicely. Brew the coffee a little stronger than you do typically.

¾ cup (180 ml) Hazelnut Milk (page 173) or store-bought hazelnut milk

½ cup (120 ml) strong-brewed coffee, or 2 shots espresso

Warm the hazelnut milk using a milk frother, or gently warm it over medium heat to your desired temperature. Pour into a mug and stir in the coffee.

Alternatively, let the coffee cool fully, then combine the cold coffee and cold hazelnut milk in an ice-filled glass for a delicious iced latte.

YIELD

1½ SERVINGS

NUTRITIONAL ANALYSIS

PER SERVING (1 CUP, OR 240 ML):

70 CALORIES

4G FAT

3G PROTEIN

1G CARBOHYDRATE

1G DIETARY FIBER

NOTE

Homemade hazelnut milk also makes a great coffee creamer, if you tend to be an Americano drinker. Use standard coffee and add a few tablespoons (about 45 ml) of hazelnut milk for a delicious hazelnut flavor.

ADD IT!

If you like your coffee drinks on the sweet side, add 1 or 2 Medjool dates or 1 to 2 tablespoons (10 to 20 g) date sugar when making hazelnut milk (see page 173).

ABOUT THE AUTHOR

◇ ◇ ◇

Michelle Miller is the creator of Sunkissed Kitchen (sunkissedkitchen.com) and BlissfullyLowCarb.com, where she shares healthy, whole foods recipes, perfect for anyone looking to improve their health or feed their family more nutritious meals.

She lives in Oregon with her rambunctious kindergartener, who is equal parts inspiration and chaos.

When she's not in the kitchen crafting beautiful meals, she's out running trails or soaking in the high desert sun.

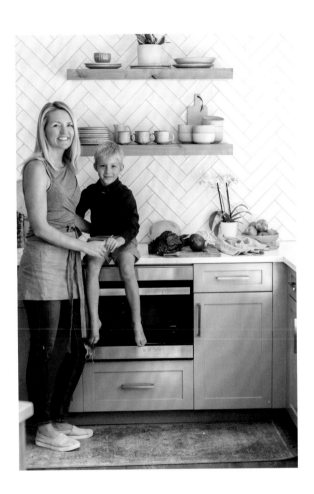

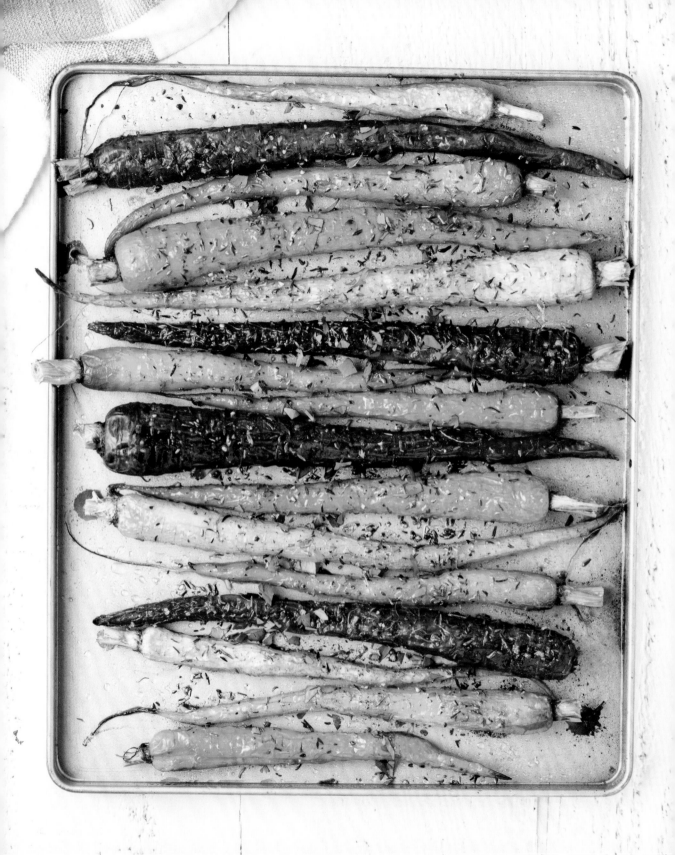

INDEX